From Patient Data to

The Principles and Practice of Health Informatics

To Ailsa and Ewan

In real life a mathematical proposition is never what we want. We make use of mathematical propositions only in making inferences from propositions that do not belong to mathematics to other propositions that likewise do not belong to mathematics.

Wittgenstein Tractatus Logico-philosophicus

From Patient Data to Medical Knowledge

The Principles and Practice of Health Informatics

Paul Taylor

Centre for Health Informatics and Multiprofessional Education (CHIME)
University College London, Archway Campus, Highgate Hill
London, N19 5LW

Blackwell
Publishing

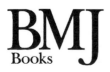

© 2006 by Blackwell Publishing Ltd
BMJ Books is an imprint of the BMJ Publishing Group Limited, used under licence

Blackwell Publishing, Inc., 350 Main Street, Malden, Massachusetts 02148-5020, USA
Blackwell Publishing Ltd, 9600 Garsington Road, Oxford OX4 2DQ, UK
Blackwell Publishing Asia Pty Ltd, 550 Swanston Street, Carlton, Victoria 3053, Australia

First published 2006

Library of Congress Cataloging-in-Publication Data
Taylor, P. (Paul), Dr.
   From patient data to medical knowledge : the principles and practice of health
informatics / Paul Taylor.
       p. ; cm.
   Includes bibliographical references and index.
   ISBN-13: 978-0-7279-1775-1 (alk. paper)
   ISBN-10: 0-7279-1775-7 (alk. paper)
   1. Medical informatics.
       [DNLM: 1. Medical Informatics. 2. Public Health Informatics. WA 26.5 T245p 2006]
I. Title.

   R858.T35 2006
   610.285—dc22   2005031692
ISBN-13: 978 0 7279 1775 1
ISBN-10: 0 7279 1775 7

A catalogue record for this title is available from the British Library

Set in 9.5/12pt Meridien by SPI Publisher Services, Pondicherry, India
Printed and bound in India by Replika Press Pvt. Ltd, Harayana

Commissioning Editor: Mary Banks
Editorial Assistant: Ariel Vernon
Development Editor: Nick Morgan
Production Controller: Debbie Wyer

For further information on Blackwell Publishing, visit our website:
http://www.blackwellpublishing.com

The publisher's policy is to use permanent paper from mills that operate a sustainable
forestry policy, and which has been manufactured from pulp processed using acid-free and
elementary chlorine-free practices. Furthermore, the publisher ensures that the text paper
and cover board used have met acceptable environmental accreditation standards.

Contents

Acknowledgements

I would like to thank my friends and colleagues at CHIME, especially David Ingram and Jeannette Murphy. I also owe a significant debt to John Fox who introduced me to the field. The other alumni of the Advanced Computation Laboratory have been an enormous influence. I have learned a great deal from the students of the UCL Graduate Programme in Health Informatics, among whom Chris Martin stands out as a friend and collaborator. Finally, above all I must thank Jean McNicol. I could not have written this without her support, encouragement and understanding.

About this book

The best way to learn about a subject, I now realise, is to write a book about it. Another good way is to teach it. In 1999, University College London (UCL) started a postgraduate programme in Health Informatics. As the programme director it was largely my responsibility to define the curriculum, a somewhat daunting task in a new and ill-defined subject. I decided, early on, that students should take an introductory module that would give them a grounding in the necessary theory and would also provide a survey of the different problems and applications that make up the field of Health Informatics. The module was called 'Principles of Health Informatics'. But what are the principles of Health Informatics?

The course, and the introductory module, has now run five times. Our students are all part-time and mostly work in information or clinical roles in the National Health Service (NHS) or other health care organisations (we recruit a small number of international students). They have brought with them a wealth of experience and practical intelligence. Each year I have presented the introductory module in a different way and each year the students have responded to some aspects and not to others. As a result, over the years, my feeling for what the essence of Health Informatics is has changed. Eventually it developed to the point where I felt my understanding of what mattered could be set out in a short book that could serve as a text for our course and for other similar courses.

Writing the book has been complicated by the fact that the UK government is in the process of pushing through an unprecedented programme of investment in information technology, which has raised the profile of the field and also introduced some new and quite specific challenges. I have tried to deal with these, while recognising that specific agenda may well have moved on again by the time this book comes to press. The field is inevitably a rapidly changing one.

The book has three parts. Part 1 consists of an introductory chapter and three further chapters, each of which deals with one of the 'grand challenges' I identify for Health Informatics. This part provides a broad introduction to the field of Health Informatics. Part 2 deals with various techniques used in Health Informatics and the theory behind some of them. A key element of this is the question of how we can represent clinical concepts in computer programs such as electronic health care records or decision support systems. I argue that many applications of Health Informatics can be seen as drawing on techniques from computer science that, in turn, are based on logic. I therefore provide a brief introduction to logic and then to subjects that, in some sense, involve the application of logic: controlled clinical terminology, knowledge representation, ontologies and clinical standards. By way of a contrast I also discuss probability, in two chapters, one of which deals with decision making and the other with statistics, an element in research but also in machine learning and data mining. Part 3 explores attempts to apply Health Informatics in practice. This includes a chapter on theories of organisational change and two further chapters: one dealing with attempts to change clinical practice by improving the dissemination of information and the other on the change management issues raised by attempts to introduce new technology into health care organisations. I also offer some closing thoughts in a final concluding chapter.

I hope that the book will be of interest to anyone who has cause to think about how we use information in health care, and I have tried not to make assumptions of any form of prior knowledge about information, IT, computer science or health care. I live and work in the UK and the overwhelming majority of my students have been employees of the NHS. Many of the examples I discuss are drawn from this experience. I hope, however, that the subject and the themes are nevertheless relevant to a wider audience.

Part 1
Three Grand Challenges for Health Informatics

CHAPTER 1
Introduction

Diagnosis

Diagnosis seems a good place to start a book about medicine and health care. After all, diagnosis is the first decision that a doctor has to make in the management of a new patient. What exactly do we mean by diagnosis? What is involved in diagnosing an illness? The patient arrives with a story about a problem, a complaint. The doctor first listens to the story, then starts to ask questions. Let us imagine a patient presents at accident and emergency (A&E) with acute abdominal pain and is seen by a junior doctor. As soon as the doctor hears that the patient has acute abdominal pain, he or she will start thinking of the seven or so common (or fairly common) diseases that can cause acute abdominal pain. The doctor might, later on, consider some more unlikely diagnoses as well. He or she will try to establish, through asking a set of questions and performing a simple set of examinations, what the patient's symptoms are.

The trick in diagnosis is to work out, given the symptoms, what the disease is. Or at least what the disease probably is. Or, maybe, what the management should be, given the relative likelihood of a number of possible diagnoses, some more sinister than others. It is, inevitably, a matter of probabilities. As it happens, probability theory gives us a simple equation for dealing with probabilities of this type. It is called Bayes' theorem. In its simplest form, it looks like this:

$$p(D|S) = p(S|D) \times p(D)/p(S)$$

Bayes' theorem

The notation may look unfamiliar: $p(D)$ stands for the probability of a disease, which is sometimes called the prevalence, prior probability or pre-test probability of a disease; $p(S)$ stands for the probability of a symptom. The vertical bar means 'given that'. It expresses the idea that the probability of one thing happening can be altered by the occurrence of another thing. So $p(S|D)$ is the probability of symptom S given that the patient has disease D. It is, therefore, a measure of how good a symptom is as a test for a disease. On the other hand, $p(D|S)$ is the probability that a patient with symptom S will turn out to be suffering from disease D. This, if you think about it, is what the doctor is trying to work out: given these symptoms what is the most likely disease? Bayes' theorem tells him/her how to do it: *the probability that a patient with symptom*

S has disease D is given by the probability of a patient with disease D having symptom S, multiplied by the prior probability of the disease, divided by the prior probability of the symptom.

Imagine if we actually tried to diagnose using Bayes' theorem. Imagine that a group of people set out to collect data on the thousands of patients who came to their hospital with acute abdominal pain. Imagine that they worked out the prevalence of the various diseases associated with abdominal pain, the prevalence of the relevant symptoms and the probability of each of these symptoms occurring in patients with each disease. Imagine that they programmed a computer to perform the calculations, following Bayes' theorem. Diagnosis would simply be a matter of entering the patient's symptoms into the computer and waiting for the result. Wouldn't that be marvellous? You would get an objective, patient-specific, quantitative, evidence-based statement of the most likely diagnosis. Isn't that the dream that lies behind the subject of this book? Well, it isn't a dream. It was done.

AAPHelp

The first trials of the system now known as AAPHelp (AAP = acute abdominal pain) were published in the 1970s. In 1972, de Dombal *et al.* reported a study in which the system that they created achieved an accuracy of 91.8%[1]. This compared favourably with the accuracy of only 79% achieved by the most senior physician to look at the patients in the study. The junior doctors did much worse. Adams *et al.* reported, in 1986, the results of a multicentre trial involving 16 737 patients[2]. The system raised initial diagnostic accuracy from 45.6% to 65.3%. Observed mortality fell by 22%. In a later European trial the residual diagnostic error rate fell by 40%[3]. The unnecessary operation rate was cut by two-fifths. The perforation rate in appendicitis cases was cut by half. In short, the system proved an astonishing success.

Or did it? If I began to suffer from abdominal pain and staggered out of my office into the A&E department of the hospital where I work, would I benefit from this system? No. Why not? Well, because it is not in routine use in this hospital or, as far as I know, in any hospital. Why not? Well, that is a longer story than the one I have just told and one with important lessons about health care, about diagnosis, about computer systems and about all kinds of things. This book is, in part, an attempt to explain that story.

The impressive results I have quoted above were not the only findings to be published. While de Dombal *et al.* were broadcasting good news in the *British Medical Journal* (*BMJ*), another group was printing bad news in the *Lancet*: 'Computer systems based on Bayes's formula have no useful role in the diagnosis of acute abdominal pain'[4]. Others came to the same conclusion. Inevitably there was argument about the methodology of the trials, the interpretation of the results and so on. Many people felt that the system was not given a fair evaluation because clinicians saw it as a threat. Other arguments centred on the usability of the system: remember that this was a long time ago in terms of user interfaces and processing power and, indeed, in terms of the number of computers readily available in hospitals.

The team behind AAPHelp regarded themselves as pioneers. Inevitably they made a number of pragmatic decisions about which diseases to include, which data items to collect, how to perform the calculations and how to present the results. They were prepared to do the best they could and then to expose the results to empirical tests, to use the system in practice and see if it worked. The clinical evidence about the system's success is, perhaps, mixed. The verdict of history is, however, unequivocal: the system pioneered by de Dombal has not led to the development of a tool used in the management of large numbers of patients.

It is worth thinking about the reasons for the failure of such a promising project. There are many possible objections to the use of AAPHelp. Some of them are quite specific, and have to do with details of the machine's operation and the practicality of its use in a particular setting. Some are more general and would apply to all systems of this type, that is, all systems that attempt to make predictions based on statistical calculations. Other even broader criticisms would apply to almost all attempts to introduce technology into clinical practice. I want to look at some of these criticisms in the rest of this chapter and in so doing to introduce some of the challenges faced by health informatics today.

Criticisms of AAPHelp

Technology in medicine

The most general criticisms reflect concerns about the way technology is used in medicine. Many clinicians are ambivalent about new technology. A doctor who has devoted years of education and training to acquiring and refining a particular skill will inevitably be reluctant to accept a new development that seems to make all that effort redundant. This was true in 1819 when Laennec introduced the stethoscope, and it remains true today[5]. Any hostility towards, or scepticism about, new technology is not necessarily Luddite or reactionary. New technology will generally be accepted if it makes it easier for doctors or nurses to perform the services that they regard as valuable. The difficulty comes when the technology seems either to get in the way of traditional ideas of good practice or to infringe on territory that clinicians regard as requiring expert judgement. Hence, radiologists welcome new and better imaging techniques, because they realise that such developments allow them to become better radiologists. Computer software that could help them interpret X-rays, however, poses a greater challenge to their belief in the value of their own expert knowledge and their existing ways of working.

For over 160 years after the development of reliable thermometers, they were not routinely used to monitor the progress of fevers[6]. The root cause of this long delay was not a reluctance to adopt new technology but rather that the notion of fever was ill defined in the medical thinking of the time. The few studies that were attempted using thermometers failed to show a correlation between temperature and the severity of other symptoms because the researchers had a unitary notion of fever. It was only when researchers developed a classification of distinct fevers that the thermometer became indispensable.

AAPHelp was a particularly problematic system for clinicians. It did not provide the physician with additional information about the patient as a thermometer or a positron emission tomography (PET) scanner does. Most medical technology aims to help the physician by revealing otherwise inaccessible information about the patient's state. The physician's expert judgement is helped by such technology and his or her decisions are better informed. AAPHelp is different. It takes the same information that the physician has, but does something different with it and then confronts him or her with the result. One of the lessons that system designers have had to learn, given the reception of AAPHelp and many similar projects, is that computer systems are most likely to be accepted if they are designed to complement clinical expertise. Decision support systems are now commonplace but the most successful ones are very different from AAPHelp. Computer aids have proved most effective in other decisions; e.g. in prescribing or in generating reminders or alerts[7]. There have been relatively few, if any, successful attempts to apply decision support to diagnostic decisions.

There are other objections to the use of technology in medicine. People are suspicious of it because they feel that it makes medicine cold and impersonal. Clinicians and their patients generally believe that medicine needs a human touch, that patients have to be treated as individuals and that an understanding of the social context and background to a case is often important. The writers of television dramas and hospital-based soap operas clearly believe that their viewers prefer doctors who connect with their patients at an emotional level. A number of health informatics interventions, notably certain attempts to provide telemedicine via videoconferencing, have foundered on the failure to recognise that a medical consultation is not just an occasion for the transfer of patient data and medical advice but is also a social encounter in which the participants have established roles and expectations. Technology that is suspected of dehumanising the consultation is often rejected. But this is not always the case. Patients sometimes express a preference for more technical interventions, perhaps believing that they result in better outcomes (see, e.g. Wallace et al.[8]). Such is the penetration of computers elsewhere that many people would be a little surprised if their doctor did not have a computer on his or her desk.

Statistical approaches to decision support
The second class of criticisms concerns the use of what we might call statistical, probabilistic or Bayesian techniques. The controversy about AAPHelp can be seen as part of a wider debate that has its roots in an anxiety about the extent to which medical practice is truly scientific. In the early post-war years,

the accepted view of the role of science in medicine held that the physician was an artisan with a scientific education; a skilled practitioner who understood and applied scientific knowledge but did so using the intuition and experience and skill required to treat unique patients. By the 1970s, however, the editorials of influential clinical journals had begun to argue that there were fundamental problems with this, and to use the term 'scientific' to describe how medicine should be practised. It was argued that medical practice was not the application of a science that is located elsewhere but was, or should be, itself a scientific activity.

Of course, the assertion that medical practice should be more scientific in character can be used to support more contentious proposals. Berg identifies two distinct views of what scientific medicine might be[9]. On one side writers argued for the standardisation of terminology, more rigorous and better structured history taking and the use of flow charts and decision tables to guide diagnostic reasoning. Medicine, on this view, is not an art informed by scientific knowledge but is itself a scientific process in which questions are defined, data collected, recorded, analysed and used to test hypotheses. On the other side were those, like de Dombal, who argued that humans were simply unable to carry out the task of diagnosis with the precision that could be achieved by mathematical tools. The limitations of short-term memory mean that we cannot retrieve and hold in our minds all the necessary facts. We are unable to see all the information that is present in the data, and intuition is hopelessly flawed when it comes to performing probabilistic computations.

Both sides argued for the introduction of new tools and new ways of thinking, but took very different approaches. The kinds of tools that de Dombal and others developed were sharply criticised by opponents who argued that the apparent rationality of statistical methods was deceptive. The messy reality of actual clinical practice meant that countless compromises, pragmatic judgements and unwarranted assumptions had to be made in the design and application of Bayesian systems. Furthermore, the output of such systems – a set of statistical scores – was alien to clinical thinking because the conclusions could not readily be interpreted as an explanation of the salient details in the patients' history.

In the three decades that have followed the development of AAPHelp, two distinct strands of research in decision support can be traced: one is the development of increasingly sophisticated approaches to the use of probabilities in clinical decision making; the other is the attempt to model the logical rules used in making decisions. Many researchers have argued that we should not attempt to build Bayesian systems, in part because in all but a few cases we do not have the required statistical data[10]. Many successful decision support systems have been built using sets (sometimes very small sets) of relatively simple logical rules that can be incorporated into electronic patient record systems or prescribing systems to perform tasks such as checking for allergies or drug interactions[7]. A great deal of the work described in this book aims to provide enhanced patient record systems that will be able to give exactly this kind of support. Much of it draws on work in computer science on the representation of knowledge, and much of that work is, in turn, ultimately based on logic.

Not all work in health informatics is underpinned by logic or probability: e.g. work in telemedicine or on the design of user-friendly websites for the general public. But most of the systems discussed in this book attempt to represent information, either about patients or about medicine. Some of these representations use sets of symbols to represent facts and the relationships between facts. Others depend on numbers, on probabilistic calculation rather than logical inference.

The use of statistical methods to support clinical decision making remains controversial. Clinicians are trained to deal with patients as individuals, whereas probabilistic calculations deal with populations. Most doctors, like most other people, find the mathematics of probability difficult. Practising clinicians have been shown to come to dramatically incorrect conclusions when asked to assess clinical information expressed in terms of mathematical probabilities[11]. But as medical knowledge advances in the post-genomic era we will learn more and more about the genetic basis for disease, and much of what we learn will be about susceptibility and risk. Already we know enough about the risk factors for certain cancers and for cardiovascular disease to mean that the effective communication of information about risk is a key component of preventative medicine. It is not easy to convey an accurate idea of risk: one study has reported that educated American women massively overestimated the incidence of breast cancer, believing that they had a 1:10 chance of dying of it within 10 years when the true likelihood was about 1:200. The development of effective tools for communicating information about risk is a fertile area of research in health informatics.

Collecting and analysing patient data

The final class of criticisms of AAPHelp deals with specific features of the system's operation. There is only one we need to look at here: the use made of patient data. Consider the processes involved in creating and using a system such as AAPHelp. The first step is to collect the data from which the statistics will be calculated. You might think this is easy enough, simply a matter of trawling through the notes and counting up how many times a patient with symptom X turned out to be suffering from disease Y. Well, not quite. Say symptom X is not mentioned in the notes. Does that necessarily mean the patient did not have the symptom? You cannot be sure. The only way to ensure that the statistics accurately reflect the symptoms and diseases of the patients is to collect all the data prospectively. Worse, it is also necessary to set out in advance exactly what questions are to be asked and how the answers are to be recorded. The process of data collection requires the standardisation not just of the set of data items to be recorded for each patient but also the terms used to record patient history. This will inevitably change the way patients are interviewed and managed. de Dombal described his method thus:

> First we created a long list with the items mentioned in the literature. Then we got rid of those items the majority of our clinical colleagues wouldn't do or where they could not agree on the method of elicitation. The reproducibility of the item is important: we have thrown out typifications of the pain as 'boring', 'burning', 'gnawing', 'stabbing'. They haven't gone because people don't use them, they've gone because people can't say what they are .... Another example which fell off was back pain with straight leg raising: an often mentioned sign. But nobody agrees on what they are talking about. What should the result of the test be? A figure? The angle the leg makes with the table? ... We could not get a group of rheumatologists, orthopedic surgeons and general practitioners to agree about what they should call 'straight leg raising' so we abandoned that.[9]

The need for a robust and well-defined set of data items to use in the Bayesian calculations clearly biases the process of history taking. If you cannot agree on how a term should be defined, it cannot go on the form. And if the term is not on the form, it is not in the history, it is not on the record and it is not available to help make a diagnosis. This is one of the most commonly remarked observations on failings of Bayesian systems; critics argue that the 'soft' data items that tend to be dropped are often the most important. Stripping out subjective impressions or observations that have to be understood in terms of a social context deprives the patient history of much of its human character and that obviously worries physicians. Human beings are able to use language to communicate pretty well – most of the time. With computers, things are very different. Although we get by, using words that have no clear, crisp definition, as soon as a computer is introduced into the process things begin to break down.

Of course there is a counter-critique: one could argue that the fact that people cannot agree on the meaning of a particular term raises questions about its value in clinical reasoning. One of the interesting conclusions reached in the work of de Dombal and others was that much of the improvement in performance that followed the introduction of AAPHelp was actually due not to the information that the statistical calculation provided but to the use of a standard data entry form that the computer system required clinicians to use in collecting the history[4]. In order for AAPHelp to generate a prediction, someone had to enter the patient's symptoms into the computer. They had to be collected in a standard format, to match the data stored in the computer. In order to manage the process efficiently, a form was designed that took the doctor through a standard set of questions. Doctors had to sit down with patients and spend between 5 and 20 min going through a checklist of the questions that all doctors know must be asked of such patients but that some of them sometimes forget. Many people believed that at least some of the improvement attributed to the software was due to the use of the form rather than the computer-generated predictions. Certainly the team accepted that the standardisation of both terminology and the process of history taking was valuable.

One conclusion that the project team drew from the experience was that 'databases do not travel'. Part of the reason doctors in different sites had different perceptions of the value of the system was that it performed better in some places than in others. There are, perhaps surprisingly, real differences in the ways clinicians define even the most obvious symptoms and even the best understood diseases. These differences again reflect underlying differences in geography, economics and organisational norms. A system that depends on the capacity of a clinical user to record a history in a standard way will run into difficulties as soon as it is moved into a setting where the users are poorly trained, trained in a different way or simply unfamiliar with the assumptions built into the design of the system. The prior probability that a patient with acute abdominal pain has appendicitis is not the same for a patient who turns up at A&E and another who is referred to the chest ward. Equally, if you install the system in a rural hospital in the north of England, you will get a different mix of patients to those seen in an urban hospital in East London. If the senior clinician in the unit is supportive of the system, it will be used in the management of different kinds of patient than will be the case if the senior clinician is reluctant to get involved.

The predictions generated by AAPHelp would be sensitive to changes, because the data the system uses to calculate the probabilities are specific to the place in which the data were collected. We should be careful about the meanings we attribute to clinical data. They carry information not just about patients but also about the time and place in which they were recorded. They are moulded by all sorts of things, from the internal politics of the institution to the social geography of the surrounding population. Crucially, they are products of the organisational processes through which they were collected.

Scientific medicine and the description of experience

At the heart of the controversy about statistical systems is a question about what use we can make of patient data, other than as an element in the patient's story. How can we capture what we need to record about a patient's signs and symptoms in terms that allow us to use them as the raw material of calculations that will inform the care of future patients? The interesting point, if we relate this back to the controversy between the Bayesians and their opponents who advocated a scientific but not a statistical approach to diagnosis, is that the standardisation of terminology and the structured recording of patient histories were first put forward by members of the second camp. And, actually, the difficulties involved in attempting to impose rigid definitions on the terms used to describe clinical conditions crop up all the time in 'scientific' medicine. The point is illustrated diagrammatically in Figure 1.1.

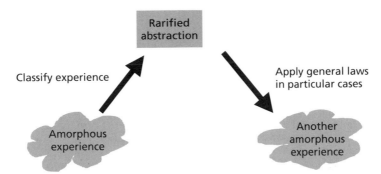

Figure 1.1 Learning from experience involves abstraction.

The goal of most quantitative clinical research is to cast observations about a patient's experience in terms that allow a connection to the experience of other patients. This involves abstraction. It involves extracting something from a messy, complicated, amorphous, individual story that is sufficiently clear and well defined to serve as the raw material of scientific study. It will involve a task not unlike that which confronted the doctors using the AAPHelp system who had to characterise their patients' pain as chronic, acute or cholicky. It will be a matter of putting pegs that are never entirely round or exactly square into holes that are either one thing or the other.

What have we learnt?

How would we do things differently now, 30 years later? What kind of system might we envisage to support a junior doctor in A&E at the start of the twenty-first century? Perhaps the most obvious difference between a new tool and the one developed by de Dombal *et al.* would be the hardware we would use. A&E departments are complex, flexible and busy environments. We would therefore perhaps want to deliver a system on a hand-held computer connected via a wireless network, something that was certainly not possible for de Dombal. What information might we expect the doctor to obtain from the system? We would be interested in three distinct types of information:

1 About the patient – we would want to provide the doctor with the fullest possible access to the patient's record, not just access to notes about previous visits to A&E or previous investigations carried out in the hospital but also his or her general practitioner's (GP's) record, and summarised information about current prescriptions, known allergies and other relevant episodes.

2 About the hospital's facilities and procedures – the doctor should be able to consult relevant guidelines, protocols and care pathways to find out about the availability of beds, theatre slots and also be able to order investigations and issue prescriptions electronically.

3 On clinical evidence and published research – the doctor might consult estimates of the extent to which genetic and environmental factors predisposed patients towards certain illnesses.

Evidence-based medicine

In recent years a movement has grown within medicine, arguing that the pace of change in medical research demands that clinicians should consult the scientific evidence before deciding about the treatment of individual patients. This is simply the most recent expression of the anxiety that sparked off the debate about Bayesian statistics – the belief that too much clinical decision making is arbitrary and idiosyncratic. Its proponents do not think it is enough that the latest advances are taught in medical schools or as part of clinicians' continuing education. If patients are to reap the benefits of new research, they believe clinicians must get into the habit of actively looking for clinical evidence when making decisions about diagnosis and management. This movement is known as 'evidence-based' medicine.

The challenge of evidence-based medicine is to treat each patient as an individual while interpreting his or her unique experience in the light of what has been learned from the experience of others. The project of health informatics – and the subject of this book – is to build tools that maximise the benefits of abstracting from the particular while minimising the costs. Evidence-based medicine is about moving from the abstract to the particular, applying clinical evidence to the amorphous experience of individual patients. Health informatics attempts to support both steps in the process: the creation of evidence out of data, and the application of evidence in the management of patients.

Health informatics and evidence-based medicine

Figure 1.2 is an attempt to illustrate the process by which patient data are transformed into clinical evidence. Three stages are identified. In the first, the data are created. It is worth clarifying the claim that is being made here. Data are not just waiting to be gathered, collected or recorded. Data are created. Recording patient history is not a simple matter of writing down observed facts. The observations emerge from the conversation between the clinician and the patient; they are a product of that conversation and take their meaning from it. Similarly when data are transmitted from one professional to another as the patient moves from primary care to an acute hospital, they alter. Patient histories are continually resummarised, recontextualised and recreated. Even the simplest statements will be reinterpreted in the light of new information, new possibilities and changing priorities.

The process of care comes to a conclusion, if treatment is successful, when the patient stops being a patient and returns to being an active healthy individual. But that is not necessarily the end of the story for the data. The details that have been recorded in the management of this patient are coded

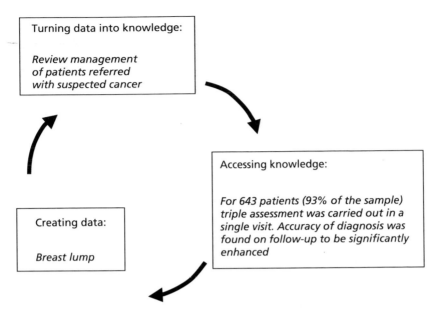

Figure 1.2 Three stages in a 'virtuous circle' of health knowledge management.

and classified to compile statistics about the management of patients with this disease, at this institution, in this region, and used to answer a range of questions. Clinical audit, clinical research and management scrutiny all depend on data. This is the second stage in the process, the transformation of clinical data into various forms of medical knowledge.

In the third stage, the loop is closed and the knowledge obtained from the data is used to inform the management of future patients. Again, the ideal of evidence-based medicine is that the essence of the aggregated data about past patients provides the empirical basis for decisions about current and future ones.

This book

The AAPHelp system attempted to do exactly that: to use data about past patients to inform the treatment of current and future patients. It attempted to complete all three arcs of the circle shown in Figure 1.2. This book describes other, more recent systems, techniques and ideas that also aim to realise the potential of IT to improve the flow of information around that circle.

The argument of this book is that the creation of systems to support clinical work has proved harder than de Dombal and other pioneers envisaged. Most medical researchers, in other fields, devote their professional lives to work that promises at best an incremental improvement in how one disease is managed or treated. Researchers in health informatics believed that they could achieve a step-change in the accuracy of diagnosis and efficacy of treatment across a swathe of common conditions. It is the scale of that potential gain rather than the track record of success that continues to motivate work in the field.

The three stages in the graphic correspond to the three 'grand challenges' for health informatics, the three generic tasks involving health information. Chapters 2–4 address each of these in turn.

References

1. de Dombal FT, Leaper DJ, Staniland JR, McCann AP, Horrocks JC. Computer-aided diagnosis of acute abdominal pain. *BMJ* 1972;2:9–13.
2. Adams ID, Chan M, Clifford PC. Computer-aided diagnosis of acute abdominal pain: a multicentre study. *BMJ* 1986;293:800–804.
3. de Dombal FT, de Baere H, van Elk PJ, *et al.* Objective medical decision making: acute abdominal pain. In: Beneken EW, Thévenin V, eds. *Advances in Biomedical Engineering*. Amsterdam, The Netherlands: IOS Press, 1993:65–87.
4. Sutton GC. How accurate is computer-aided diagnosis? *Lancet* 1989;2(8668): 905–908.
5. Reiser SJ. *Medicine and the Reign of Technology*. Cambridge: Cambridge University Press, 1978.
6. Worth-Eskes J. Quantitative observations of fever and its treatment before the advent of short clinical thermometers. *Med Hist* 1991;35:189–216.
7. Hunt DL, Haynes RB, Hanna SE, Smith K. Effects of computer-based clinical decision support systems on physician performance and patient outcomes: a systematic review. *JAMA* 1998;280(15):1339–1346.
8. Wallace P, Haines A, Harrison R, *et al.* Joint teleconsultations (virtual outreach) versus standard outpatient appointments for patients referred by their general practitioner for a specialist opinion: a randomised trial. *Lancet* 2002;359(9322): 1961–1968.
9. Berg M. *Rationalizing Medical Work*. Cambridge, MA: MIT Press, 1997.
10. Fox J, Das S. *Safe and Sound*. Cambridge, MA: MIT Press, 2000.
11. Gigerenzer G. *Reckoning with Risk: Learning to Live with Uncertainty*. London: Penguin Books, 2003.

CHAPTER 2

Reading and writing patient records

This book is concerned with the effective use of patient data: the facts, findings, measurements, observations and assessments that doctors and nurses record about the patients in their care. The creation, organisation, management and maintenance of patient records are the central preoccupations of health informatics. Indeed, the project of health informatics is often identified with the creation of an electronic integrated care record. This, it is said, will lead to a promised land in which every relevant fact about a patient will be instantly accessible, 24 h a day, 7 days a week, to his or her GP in Surbiton, cardiologist at the Royal Brompton or even to the A&E registrar in Chamonix.

The creation of such a system is not just a matter of transferring information from paper records to computer files but also requires the solution of a host of other technical, intellectual and organisational problems. There are difficulties connected with the merging of information that is currently stored in very different forms on different systems. GPs and hospitals use different systems, and often each hospital department will have a separate system. Merging information does not only mean connecting the machines on which the data is stored; the applications running on those machines must be able to communicate with each other. There are problems to do with the way information is represented in order to make it accessible to different systems and different users. There are also problems to do with security and confidentiality. How can users on different sites be identified as having a legitimate interest in a particular patient's data? How can it be verified that the patient has given consent for his or her data to be used in this way?

A clearer assessment of the potential benefits of such a system, as well as of the difficulties and risks involved in its creation, requires an understanding of the nature of a patient record, and its part in supporting patient care.

Patient-centred records

At the beginning of the twentieth century most hospitals kept patients' records in bound volumes. Entries were made when patients were seen, with the result that passages dealing with different visits of the same patient were scattered throughout the volumes. As hospitals became larger and more complex, it became necessary to allocate each patient a document or a folder that would be shared between the clinicians responsible for a patient. In 1907, new patients registering at the Mayo Clinic were assigned a number. All subsequent medical information and correspondence was filed under the patient's registration number and kept in wooden filing cabinets, accessible to all the Mayo physicians[1]. The records were no longer the private observations of a single physician but became what we would now call a patient-centred narrative.

This must rank as a pivotal moment in the prehistory of health informatics: a major advance in the capacity of the record to support patient care, achieved by means of a major redesign of that record. It is interesting to consider the physical and organisational changes that it required. One of the most significant facts about the computer age is that information can be manipulated without radically changing the physical medium on which it is stored. Before computers, ensuring that all the data an institution held on a patient were kept in one place meant rearranging bits of paper. Of course, it was not the move to storing paper in a folder rather than a book that was important but what this meant for the information itself. If we were now to carry out an analogous reorganisation, in an attempt to ensure that all the data the NHS holds on each patient are kept in one place, the fact that much of the information is stored on computers ought to make the task simpler. In some ways it is probably harder, since the computer systems in question were not designed to support the sharing of information in this way.

The reorganisation of the information also meant that the clinicians had to change the way they worked. The system crucially required that there be a single central facility from which each clinician would collect a record and to which they would return it. Dr Plummer, the architect of the original Mayo Clinic, is credited with the invention of the 'pneumatic tube', a device allowing the rapid transmission of documents around a building, and making it practical for different physicians to share a single central record store. Even in this age of intranets and email, the Mayo Clinic has not abandoned its pneumatic tube system but has upgraded it and added an extensive computer-controlled electric track, which can transport containers with up to 11 kg loads both horizontally and vertically around the building. The system now makes around 2400 trips a day, equivalent to 17 full-time messengers carrying laboratory specimens, medical records, X-rays and mail. When the Mayo Clinic's expansion is completed, it will have nearly 15 240 m of track and carry out more than 20 000 transactions a day[2].

Problem-oriented patient records

A second pivotal moment in the history of patient records is the publication in 1968 of Larry Weed's landmark paper 'Medical records that guide and teach'[3]. Consider the fragment of a medical record shown in Figure 2.1. The patient's story is told as a simple linear narrative, events are described in highly abbreviated statements arranged in a chronological order and a short paragraph for each relevant date. For the first five entries the information is set down in a way that might have seemed logical to the author but which gives no real assistance to the reader trying to make sense of the various observations. There is, however, a dramatic change at 10/2–6 pm, the end of

9/10
Pt. received 40 units of regular insulin yest. because of B & 4+ urine sugars. Got 2000 cc Amigen yest. & 500 cc D₅W. Was febrile all night up to 40 at 8 PM this gradually came down to 39. 8 PM yest. suctioned & coughed up c̄ return of ½ cup of thick white sputum – cultured also blood cultures. Was in must. tent c̄ mucomist overnight. At 4 PM yest had B-R base. Sputum smear unremarkable – WBC's but no bacteria.

9/10-12:30
10 o'clock urine 2-3+/0. Given 10 U. reg. ins. at 12:30 PM. Temp. down to 38? Suctioned N.T. ō little return. However during suctioning pt. vomited 100-150 cc green fluid. Proximal jejunostomy tube draining well now.

9/11-9 AM
Urine 3+ given 10 U reg. insulin. Pt. was hiccuping all night & this AM. Levine tube passed c̄ 900-1000 cc bileous fluid removed. Jejunostomy tubes have been draining minimally. Will have Levine tube down.

(THREE PAGES OF SIMILAR NOTES FOLLOW UNTIL 9/26/67)

9/26
Last night 10PM had seizure like behavior and acting strange. Apparently hallucinating. Blood sugar didn't register on destrostix. Had been given 10 units reg. insulin at 8 PM after IV glucose returned to nl. This AM vomited up brown black fluid 300 cc + for occult blood. NG tube had been out since 5 PM yest. NG tube replaced & some material small amt. withdrawn. Pt. now NPO ō NG. tube to Gomco.

9/27
Still febrile – Ampicillin 1 g qid – continued; Blood cult. drawn to check if septicemia still present. Chest x-ray still present. Chest x-ray today shows infiltrate in (R) lower lobe. No effusion. Sputum grew out pseudomonas but Dr. _____ elected not to treat this.
ON SERVICE NOTE (please read revised problem list and please use #'s shown)

10/2-6 PM
#1 Chronic Relapsing Panc.:
  b. *Diabetes:* will continue moment-to-moment Rx of spot urines for now. Today c̄ only 10 U regular insulin pt. spilling mainly 2-3+.
    Plan: BLD sugar tomorrow
  c. *Panc. insuff.:* will begin Cotazyn-B
#2 Complications Following Laparotomy:
  c. *Post op ileus:* KUB tomorrow. Pt. now tolerating ice cream and occ. candy. bs. poor; s gross distention; stool passes regularly ⟶ fistula

Imp: prob. resolving now
Plan: KUB and continue small feedings
d. *Sepsis:* afebrile now on Ampicillin. see flow sheet. Reculture tomorrow.
b. *RLL Pneumonia:* Film of 9/28 shows some ↑ in this process. Will repeat P.A. chest tomorrow & cultures.
e. *Colonic-Cutaneous Fistula:* Continues to drain semi-formed stool several times per day; the problem is that stool drains onto granulating abd. wound.
  Plan: culture stool; Remove some non-func stay sutures; Freq dressings & consider colostomy bag for fistula

10/3
#1 Chronic Relapsing Panc.:
  c. *Panc. insufficiency:* Cotazyn-B will be begun (special purchase) and will evaluate effect on absorption and/or stool content by measuring amt of fat
  f. *Pain:* pt. still requires freq narcotics. Neurosurg will eventually perform epidural block and depending upon results will consider cordotomy
#2 Complications Following Laparotomy:
  b. *RLL Pneumonia:* Chest x-ray today shows marked resolution of previously described infiltrates; pt. has been afebrile – sputum recultured (see #2d).
  c. *Post op ileus:* KUB today shows little improvement from film of 9/29. Ba in same position in colon which is distal to fistula. Despite this x-ray findings will continue to feed (see #2f). Bowel sounds poor and abd. seems slightly more distended. Will give oil retention enema to try to clear distal colon.
  d. *Sepsis:* Pt. has been afebrile, cultures repeated today; ō (M) heard today; has been on Ampicillin x 9 days. Although potential still present this problem is under relatively good control.
  e. *Colonic-Cutaneous Fistula:* all stay sutures removed today and wound is well granulated but constantly bathed c̄ stool. Colostomy bag applied to try to control this drainage. Etiology of fistula? but may be serving decompressive function.
  f. *Malnutrition:* Total protein = 6.1 c 2.1/4.0 = A/G in 1965. Wt. has ↓ from 141# ⟶ 113# since adm.
    Imp: little resolution of ileus, in fact. most of food stays in stomach probably; this remains the main problem; other as above fairly well controlled except malnutrition.
    Plan: as above plus give gastro-graffin per NG tube and watch progress; *avoid surgery.*

Figure 2.1 Sequence of notes extracted from a complicated record. In the first unstructured portion, facts and phrases are presented that suggest difficulties in many systems, but the confusion in such a tangle of illogically grouped bits of information is such that one cannot reliably discern how (or if) the physician defined and logically pursued each problem. From [3] with permission. Copyright © 1968 Massachusetts Medical Society.

the first column. After this, whenever the record is updated, the observations are organised according to a list of the problems involved in the management of this patient. This list of 'currently active problems' provides an organising structure for the record. The effect of the transformation is striking.

The idea behind the problem-oriented record is simple but powerful: clinicians should structure their observations using a list of the patient's current problems. Each time they need to make a decision about a problem, they can consult the record and find the information they require organised under headings that reflect their approach to the patient's management. The idea became associated with the acronym SOAP, so that for each problem the clinician was supposed to record observations under four headings: Subjective (what the patient says); Objective (what the doctor sees and hears); Assessment (what the doctor thinks); and Plan (what is to be done).

It is instructive, at this distance, to read Weed's original paper. It starts:

> The beginning clinical clerk, the house officer and practising physician are all confronted with conditions that are frustrating in every phase of

medical action. The purpose of this article is to identify and discuss these conditions and point out solutions. To deal effectively with these frustrations it will be necessary to develop a more organised approach to the medical record, a more rational acceptance and use of medical personnel and a more positive attitude about the computer in medicine.

Weed recognised that adding an extra element to the way medical information was recorded would involve extra work unless new tools were available to help with the task: i.e. computerised tools. Later in the article he writes: 'It would seem most logical to have the physician enter the problem statements directly onto the computer.' Indeed, given how long ago all this happened, and how little progress there was in the computerisation of patient records during the 1970s, 1980s and even the 1990s, it is quite surprising to discover the extent to which Weed's paper builds on the pioneering work done by Warner Slack *et al.* on computer-based medical history systems[4]. This work was published as long ago as 1966 (it will be a theme of this book that health informatics is a field in which promises and expectations are renewed more often than they are fulfilled).

Although the problem-based medical record is still taught in medical schools, and still talked about, the tools that Weed recognised as being essential for organising patient information in this way did not appear as he expected. Despite the promising results of Slack *et al.*, it proved harder than anyone had expected to get computers onto physicians' desks and to get patient records onto the hard disks of those computers. In the UK in the 1970s, and even the 1980s, the debate was not about moving from paper to computer-based records but about moving from Lloyd George envelopes to A4 folders[5].

Computer support for problem-oriented records

In order to understand what was problematic about the move to computers, we need to think about what information a computer system to support problem-oriented patient records would require. First, the clinician must be able to record a list of problems. He or she must be able to change the status of a problem from active to inactive and, possibly, to change the order in which problems are listed. None of that seems too complicated. Next the clinician must record the set of observations that will make up the patient history.

Every observation of the patient's state is recorded in relation to a problem, but any might later need to be reinterpreted in the context of some other problem. It follows that each observation must include enough contextual information for it to be understood in relation to a different problem. Observations must therefore be recorded as sets of distinct statements that can be understood in isolation. If the record is organised around a changing list of problems, the original chronological ordering of the observations is lost, and so too is the narrative. If the reader is to make sense of the history, each observation must include some of the narrative. It is not enough to write 'node negative', or even that a physical examination concluded that the lymph nodes were not enlarged. The observation would have to state that a physical examination conducted in response to a suggested diagnosis of breast cancer concluded that the lymph nodes were not enlarged.

It does not follow that the clinician would have to type in all this information, for every observation. The computer system would have to be designed so that the contextual information is recorded as part of the history and could be associated with the observation by the computer. The software designer would have to provide a template for each of the clinical contexts to be supported.

Medical ontologies

Say we are concerned with consultations in general practice. The software designer might choose to represent such consultations as a set of activities performed by a GP in respect of a patient. The designer might say that each activity has a goal and that the goal is defined in terms of a clinical question and a patient problem. Each activity also generates observations, in the form of statements about the presence or absence of signs, and then about their severity, cause and location. The designer needs to have a model for the kinds of things recorded as observations and for the kinds of things required as contextual data for the interpretation of observations. So when the software is used to make a record of a consultation, it would ask the user to record one or more activities (e.g. *physical examination*). For each activity the system would ask first for the patient problem (*breast cancer*) and the clinical question (*diagnosis*) and then for a list of observations (one of which might be *lymph node enlargement* is *absent*). The finding would be recorded within a context that contains all the additional facts with which the finding will have to be associated.

In Table 2.1 this model is set out using a formal syntax developed for computer languages. The syntax is actually very simple but the details are not important here. The important point is that it is a model of what is involved in recording a consultation; it does not embody any medical knowledge. A piece of software implementing this model would not know, or need to know, about the physiology of the lymphatic system, the anatomy of the upper body or the epidemiology of cancer. Another important point is that the model is far too simple: we have not dealt with the recording of dates, patient's name, doctor's name, levels of suspicion, management plans, provisional diagnoses, assessments and so on. The longer you think about it, the more inadequate the model seems. It would be no mean feat to design a model that is clear and simple and yet able to cope with the huge variety of encounters involved in general practice, and to reflect the varying preferences and styles of general practitioners. There are competing demands for the design of such things to be both complete and simple.

This kind of model is often called an ontology. The term 'ontology' is borrowed from a branch of philosophy concerned with questions of what kinds of thing can be said to exist. In health informatics (and computer

Table 2.1 A simple ontology for GP consultations, defined in extended Backus–Naur Form (eBNF). The symbols of BNF are as follows: '::=' means 'is defined as', | means 'or'. Items enclosed in { } may be repeated, items enclosed in [ ] are optional. Category names are enclosed within < >.

Consultation ::=
  {Activity}
Activity ::=
  Goal
  Observation list
Goal ::=
  <Patient problem>
  <Clinical question>
Observation list ::=
  {Observation}
Observation ::=
  <Finding> is present |
  <Finding> is absent
  [<Location>]
  [<Severity>]

---

science more generally) the word is used to refer to a specification of the concepts and relationships that can exist for a particular domain and application. Developing robust ontologies of medicine and clinical practice has been a major aim of many health informatics projects. Table 2.2 shows a fragment of a patient record set out using a more realistic model of the kinds of things that need to be recorded as associated data for a single test result.

Controlled clinical terminologies

Some designers of computer-based patient record systems assumed that they would have to provide their users with more than just a set of templates mapping out the structure of the things that might need to be recorded. They assumed that they would need to provide a complete standard terminology for recording clinical histories. That is to say, they would provide not only an ontology but also a list of concrete terms to fill the ontology's abstract structures: a controlled clinical terminology. It is worth pausing to reflect on the magnitude of this ambition. The proposal is not to come up with a complete list of all known diseases, suitably qualified, but rather to come up with a complete list of everything that might need to be recorded about a patient: signs, symptoms, social circumstances and so on. The benefits are obvious. A standardised vocabulary would avoid confusion and ambiguity. Eradicating synonyms, slang and shorthand would simplify the compilation of statistics. If all the required terms are known to the

Table 2.2 A single element from a patient record showing the complexity of the associated information required.

```
<ELEMENTITEM>
  <ATTRIBUTES>
  <RCUID>uk.ac.ucl.wh. anticoag.329802</RCUID>
  <ACCESSAMENDRIGHTS>AAR_CLINICAL</ACCESSAMENDRIGHTS>
  <SYNAPSESOBJECTID>INR Test.928272660000</SYNAPSESOBJECTID>
  <SYNAPSESPATIENTID>jones04-08-199815:03:08</SYNAPSESPATIENTID>
  <EHCRSOURCE>uk.ac.ucl.wh.cardiovascular.ACDATA1.MDB</EHCRSOURCE>
  <AUTHORISATIONSTATUS>ATTESTED</AUTHORISATIONSTATUS>
  <SUBJECTOFINFORMATION>PATIENT</SUBJECTOFINFORMATION>
  <HEALTHCAREACTIVITYLOCATION>Warmington Hospital, Warmington,
UK</ HEALTHCAREACTIVITYLOCATION>
  <LEGALLYRESPONSIBLEHEALTHCAREAGENT>Dr. David Dodds, Warmington Hospital,
Warmington, UK</LEGALLYRESPONSIBLEHEALTHCAREAGENT>
  <INFORMATIONPROVIDER>HAEMATOLOGY LAB</INFORMATIONPROVIDER>
  <LOCALE>en_GB</LOCALE>
  </ATTRIBUTES>
  <VALUE>
  <VALUEATTRIBUTES>
  <SOID>null</SOID>
  </VALUEATTRIBUTES>
  <NUMERIC>
  <QUANTITYVALUE>1.6</QUANTITYVALUE>
  </NUMERIC>
  </VALUE></ELEMENTITEM>
```

system designer, he or she can design a simple menu-based interface allowing the user to enter terms without typing. If the benefits are obvious, the scale of the challenge should also be apparent. In fact, even if it seems immediately obvious that this is extremely difficult, it is not until you have thought about it for a little while, and some researchers have spent years and even decades on these questions, that you come to appreciate how hard it really is.

We will come back to the business of representing clinical terminology and the role of medical ontologies in later chapters. It is worth mentioning one of the reasons why it is difficult. In 1918, the American College of Surgeons began to inspect hospitals and assess the quality of their record-keeping; as a result, in the 1920s forms were introduced in an attempt to ensure that complete records were kept of basic clinical information[6]. However, attempts to standardise what was recorded were, and remain, controversial. Doctors wanted, and still want, to decide for themselves how and what they should record, arguing that if they are to treat each patient as an individual, they must be able to treat each patient's record as different.

In the UK, Lloyd George's government required GPs who treated patients under the terms of the 1911 National Insurance act to 'keep such records as might be required of them under their conditions of service'. The aim was to gain statistical information about the health of the population. Doctors were given a tin box in which to keep the records that were to be returned at the end of each year. Although the practice was abandoned during the 1914–1918 war, the tin boxes determined the shape of GP records for the rest of the century. An attempt, after the war, to agree a standard for the record GPs should keep came up with two recommendations: the bizarrely general one that it should be a permanent record of the information required to support each patient's care, and the bizarrely specific one that it should be filed in envelopes that could be stored in cabinets designed for the old tin boxes[5]. There was to be no agreement on a standard set of data items to be recorded and hence no standard form.

If it were difficult for American hospitals and British family doctors in the 1920s to agree standard forms for recording patient encounters, how much harder must it be to get the profession to agree on a standard set of terms to describe those encounters? These difficulties are not just quibbles about terminology but reflect profound and genuine differences about the nature of diseases, the efficacy and appropriateness of interventions and the role of medical professionals. They stem from variations within and between nations and cultures, differences in training and experience as well as the priorities and prejudices of individuals.

Controlled clinical terminologies have nevertheless been developed. The International Classification of Diseases (ICD 10) is sponsored by the World Health Organization (WHO) and is used mainly to standardise the recording of diagnoses in order to compile statistics about the prevalence of diseases in populations[7]. Read Codes are a British attempt to develop a set of standard codes for use in primary care[8]. The Systematised Nomenclature of Medicine (SNOMED) is a similar initiative on the part of the College of American Pathologists. A merger of the two has created SNOMED CT, the first release of which, at the time of writing, is somewhat overdue[9]. Another project, Medical Subject Headings (MESH), created a standard set of terms for indexing biomedical research literature, and a related project, Unified Medical Language System (UMLS), attempts to provide a common structure within which MESH and the other systems can be used[10].

For many primary care physicians in the UK, the use of Read Codes to provide a standardised vocabulary for the recording at least of summary diagnoses is perhaps the most keenly felt change introduced as part of this drive towards a more structured and accessible patient record. Some research suggests that although the codes are widely used, they are not used consistently or wisely. A study of coding for diabetes in GP practices found that only one Read Code (C10, diabetes mellitus) was used in all the 17 practices studied and that it was applied to between 14% and 98% of patients with diabetes. Only 45% of diabetic patients had their type of diabetes coded[11].

Similarly, an examination of the records of 1680 patients found that only 47% of those with ischaemic heart disease could be identified by searching for the Read Code[12].

Van der Lei's first law of health informatics

We might think that medical records serve simply to support patient care, but actually they have a variety of roles. The notion of 'supporting patient care' is in any case a complex one and records have more than one purpose within it, from providing an aide memoire for an individual clinician to facilitating communication between the members of a care team. They also fulfil a number of other functions: from a legal one as the record of an encounter that may lead to litigation, a potential role in teaching and research and a source of important administrative data.

The point is brought home in a cost–benefit analysis that Wang *et al.* carried out in an attempt to assess the net financial benefit of an electronic medical record. They used an expert panel to estimate costs and benefits[13]. The estimates are shown in Table 2.3 together with a calculation of the net benefit, both in real terms and under an assumption that costs and benefits in future years are discounted at 5% per annum. For our purposes the interest is largely in the anticipated savings. Some accrue from easier access to the data: transcription costs are lowered and the costs of physically retrieving patients' records (chart pull costs) are reduced. However, most of the savings are because the system is able to carry out new functions based on the data. It is assumed that the system will save money by reminding the user of less expensive medications and by alerting him or her to possible adverse drug events (See Box 2.1). Similarly decision support would mean fewer laboratory tests and fewer radiological procedures. There would be improvements in fee-for-service reimbursement and fewer billing errors. Some of these assumptions might seem naive – experience has shown that decision support is not terribly effective in changing the behaviour of physicians – but there is clearly potential for savings.

Whether or not the estimates are optimistic, what should be clear is that the information entered onto the patient record is to be used not just for patient care but also to support other administrative and financial functions.

Using data for more than one purpose creates problems, however. Diagnosis-related groups (DRGs) are used to classify clinical cases according to criteria that reflect the cost of treating them. American hospitals use DRGs when returning records of their workload to Medicare, the agency that reimburses them for treating certain patients. Hsia *et al.* found a 20.8% error rate in the DRG coding data they looked at, and the proportion of errors favouring the hospitals (61.7%) suggested there was a significant non-random element in the process[14]. Data, as has already been discussed, are inevitably moulded by the process through which they are collected. Van der Lei has proposed a first law of health informatics that states that data should be used only for the purpose for which they are collected and that if

Table 2.3 A cost–benefit analysis for an electronic patient record (based on estimates from [13] with permission from Elsevier. © 2003 Excerpta Medica Inc.).

	Initial cost	Year 1	Year 2	Year 3	Year 4	Year 5	Total
Costs ($)							
Software license	1600	1600	1600	1600	1600	1600	
Implementation	3400						
Support	1500	1500	1500	1500	1500	1500	
Hardware	6600			6600			
Productivity loss		11 200					
Annual costs ($)	13 100	14 300	3100	9700	3100	3100	46 400
Present value of annual costs ($)	13 100	13 585	2798	8317	2525	2399	29 623
Benefits ($)							
Chart pull savings		3000	3000	3000	3000	3000	
Transcription savings		2700	2700	2700	2700	2700	
Prevented adverse drug events			2200	2200	2200	2200	
Drug savings			16 400	16 400	16 400	16 400	
Lab savings					2400	2400	
Radiology savings					8300	8300	
Charge capture					7700	7700	
Prevented billing error					7600	7600	
Annual benefits ($)		5700	24 300	24 300	50 300	50 300	154 900
Present value of annual benefits ($)		5415	21 931	20 834	40 970	38 921	128 071
Net benefit ($)	(13 100)	(8600)	21 200	14 600	47 200	47 200	121 600
Present value of net benefit ($)	(13 100)	(8170)	19 133	12 518	38 445	36 522	85 348

Note: Figures shown in parentheses are negative, i.e. occur in years where costs exceed savings.

Box 2.1 Doctor's handwriting: computerised physician order entry

Have you heard the joke about the couple called in to see their son's teacher? 'Your child has atrocious handwriting', the teacher tells them, at which the mother turns to the father and cries: 'Wonderful, I've always hoped he could be a doctor.' The idea that doctors have especially poor handwriting is an old one and it is one of those commonplaces that researchers feel driven to test. (See Balachandran and Roy for another[1].) Lyons *et al.* carried out a quantitative comparative study, deriving an 'illegibility score' from the error rate of a computerised optical character recognition system[2]. Participants were asked to provide samples of neat handwriting on which to train the system. The doctors had a higher median score – i.e. less legible handwriting – than other groups (nursing and administrative staff), taken individually or combined. Of course, although the method is admirably quantitative, the measure is indirect and it is possible that distinctive or unusual script might generate errors and yet be perfectly readable to the human eye. A more direct, albeit subjective, approach was taken by Cheeseman and Boon, who analysed entries written by doctors and by nurses in patients' notes and found significantly more illegible entries in those written by doctors[3].

It is not, however, really a laughing matter. Michigan State Representative Edward Gaffney was mistakenly given prednisone, a steroid, instead of Pravachol, a cholesterol inhibitor, and responded by introducing a bill that would make authors of illegible prescriptions liable to fines of up to $1000[4]. In 1999 an American cardiologist was fined $225 000 when a patient died after the pharmacist misread his prescription for Isordil, an antianginal drug, as a prescription for Plendil, an anti-hypertensive drug[5].

Drug name mix-ups are surprisingly common. Every year, the United States Pharmacopeia (USP) publishes a list of similar drug names that have caused mix-ups in hospitals[6]. There are thousands of entries and the problem accounts for 15% of the reports received by the USP. Interestingly, when the American Food and Drug Administration approves a new drug for the US market, it not only requires evidence about the biochemical qualities of the pharmaceutical but also carries out tests on the drug's proposed name. Both the spoken sound and written appearance of the name are tested against a database of 17 000 existing trade names using computer analysis while panels of physicians, nurses and pharmacists carry out simulations to assess confusability. Yet the problems still occur. AstraZeneca produces a drug called Seroquel for the treatment of schizophrenia. Bristol-Myers Squibb's Serzone, on the other hand, is a treatment for depression. Several patients have had to

(*continued*)

> **Box 2.1 Doctor's handwriting: computerised physician order entry** (*continued*)
>
> be admitted to hospital having received Seroquel instead of Serzone or vice versa, with symptoms including hallucination, paranoia, diarrhoea, vomiting, muscle weakness and dizziness.
>
> ## References
>
> 1. Balachandran AP, Roy SM. Quantum Anti-Zeno Paradox. *Phys Rev Lett* 2000:4019–4022.
> 2. Lyons R, Payne C, McCabe M, Fielder C. Legibility of doctors' handwriting: quantitative comparative study. *BMJ* 1998;317(7162):863–864.
> 3. Cheeseman GA, Boon N. Reputation and the legibility of doctors' handwriting in situ. *Scott Med J* 2001;46(3):79–80.
> 4. http://www.wnem.com/Global/ story.asp?S=1937955&nav=7k75Nsjz
> 5. Hughes C. Thou shalt write legibly. *BMJ* 2003;327(7413):s67–s68.
> 6. Hampton T. Similar drug names a risky prescription. *JAMA* 2004;291(16): 1948–1949.

no purpose was defined prior to collection, they should not be used[15]. The law is probably too restrictive. The gains in efficiency that result from making administrative use of data collected primarily to support patient care are too great to be ignored, but the law stands as a useful reminder of the dangers of the practice.

Narrative-based medicine

The twin issues of how to define ontologies for clinical activities and how to define a set of controlled clinical terms have dominated research into the computer-based record systems that Weed anticipated in his 1968 paper. The underlying aim of such research is to identify the appropriate structures for recording patient information. For these researchers, the need for a structure is given. There are, however, opposing voices.

It is argued by some that the essential element in the patient record is the patient's narrative and that eliciting and interpreting it should be the primary aim of the physician[16]. Clinical method, it is argued, should be recognised as an interpretive act that draws on innate narrative skills to interpret the stories told by patients. These critics also argue that interpreting narratives is not a matter of classifying and categorising the medical elements in these stories. Rather, the argument goes, practitioners might be able to listen more constructively to their patients' stories if they tried to understand them as stories, rather than attempting to express them in the structured and standardised format of the medical history. It is clear that if imposing a form of structure on the taking of a medical history is problematic, then attempting to record it in a predefined template using a standard set of terms is going to be extremely problematic.

The difficulty with using codes is not that there are not enough of them.* The problem with coding is that there are lots of things in medicine that are difficult to state precisely or that are not known unequivocally. Codes are designed expressly to strip away levels of nuance and ambiguity. Doctors, especially general practitioners, however, deal with patients whose problems are presented in an unstructured, disorganised fashion, and are not easily categorised. It is estimated that 50% of GP encounters end without a firm classification or diagnosis being reached. Problems evolve over time, and the reason the patient made the appointment often becomes clear only in retrospect. Codes inevitably fail to capture the richness of the doctor–patient communication. Even though systems such as the Read Codes do not provide fixed definitions for the terms that are included, restricting clinicians to the terms in the set may nevertheless encourage a reductionist approach, as doctors are led to fit patients into the provided categories. The 'taming' of narrative encouraged by coding has been criticised by Kay and Purves, who see the 'story stuff' as perhaps the most useful part of the record[17].

The role of the record in medical work

Berg, who considered the computer-based record from a sociological perspective, argued that the record is not simply a repository of information about a patient but also helps to shape communication between doctor and patient and is thus directly relevant to the way that patients' stories unfold[18]. As has already been discussed, data are not recorded so much as created. The initial hypothesis formed by the clinician will determine which questions are asked and help shape the answers that the patient gives. What is later recorded will be a *post hoc* rational reconstruction of the encounter. The same data will subsequently be recontextualised, resummarised and re-represented through processes adapted to the demands of medical work. We need to reflect on how an electronic patient record could be made to fit this environment, and should not assume that simply because the computer-based record is better by certain criteria it will actually work better in practice. Berg makes the important point that most information that health care professionals deal with is incomplete, ambiguous, subjective or in some ways unreliable. The aim of the information gathering recorded in patient histories is not definitively to establish the truth but to provide an adequate basis for action. For a doctor actively involved in treating a patient there is only one real problem: what best to do next.

---

*Version 3 of the Read Codes includes as one of the possible causes of injury: *Fumes from combustion of polyvinylchloride and similar material in conflagration, in convalescent home*; the list of occupations includes *Wild animal attendant* and the list of products for special diets covers 14 different shapes of pasta, one of which, spaghetti, has 12 different manufacturers, some of whom produce 2 or 3 different forms of gluten-free spaghetti, meaning that there is one term for *Glutafin GF long cut spaghetti* and another for *Glutafin GF short cut spaghetti*.

It follows from this that any proposals for building an electronic record must be grounded in a realistic conception of what medical work entails. Berg warns against the temptation to repair 'incomplete' or 'messy' records for completeness' sake, and worries that recording data in predetermined ways is too restrictive. The debate about whether or not a defined structure should be imposed on the patient record is unlikely to be resolved. The best approach will inevitably involve weighing the gains and losses of each approach on the best balance of organisation and richness of expression. The question becomes one of the appropriate levels at which to structure the record. Tange *et al.* argue that an intermediate level of 'granularity' is best for information retrieval: 'Most benefit can be expected from medical history and physical examination notes divided into organ systems and progress notes divided into problem segments'[19].

Electronic health care records

The question of granularity is of vital importance when we consider the prospect, mentioned in the opening paragraph of this chapter, of an electronic health record (EHR) that allows information to be shared between the different institutions responsible for a patient's care. One way of achieving this is to design a piece of what might be termed 'middleware', which would recast queries from one institution's computer in terms of the data structures used by another's computer. This could only be devised if the computer systems that are to be linked represent information in ways that are compatible.

A major area of research in health informatics concerns the elaboration of standards that could guide the developers of hospital and general practice information systems to make EHRs possible[20]. One way of devising the standard is to put together what computer scientists call an architecture for an EHR. An architecture does not dictate what information must be contained in a record. Nor does it say how any EHR system should be implemented. The architecture is a model of the generic features necessary in an EHR for it to be communicable and complete, retain integrity across systems, countries and time, and be a useful and effective ethico-legal record of care. The architecture is presented as a conceptual model of the information in any EHR. Models of information will be dealt with in Chapter 8.

Hospital episode statistics

The patient record is not the only place in which data about patients is recorded. Most hospitals use a Patient Administration System to store information required to manage the patient's journey through the secondary care system. This will include details of the patient's admission and discharge dates, details of outpatient appointments and A&E visits. The data are a mix of medical and administrative details, largely entered by clerical staff. Crucially there will also be a summary statement about each episode, recorded using one of the standard coding systems described above. This statement is usually recorded by a 'clinical coder', who will read case notes and discharge summaries before deciding on the appropriate classification.

In the UK this information is collated nationally. Each hospital submits monthly returns to an 'NHS-wide clearing service', which in turn provides quarterly returns to the Department of Health's Hospital Episode Statistics (HES) database. The information is used by the government to monitor activity in the NHS and inform decisions about the allocation of resources. The HES database is the most comprehensive national database of patient information. It is also used for a variety of other purposes, by various government agencies, regional and local bodies and hospital boards, and by academics and researchers. It is used for performance management and clinical governance.

The issue of clinical governance was brought to the fore by an official enquiry set up following the discovery that surgeons at Bristol Royal Infirmary had performed complex heart operations on young people over a number of years without anyone noticing that the mortality rate for these operations was a great deal worse than it should have been[21]. The enquiry noted: 'Bristol was awash with data. There was enough information from the late 1980s onwards to cause questions about mortality rates to be raised both in Bristol and elsewhere had the mindset to do so existed.'

If HES is to be analysed in detail, and without being aggregated across large numbers of trusts, and if it is to be used for a variety of purposes, it becomes more important to ensure that it is accurate. A 2002 report by the Audit Commission found that although the accuracy of coding was improving, it was still variable, and in 10% of hospitals error rates of more than 20% were found[22]. Clinical coders are often poorly trained, clinicians are often not involved in the process of coding and adequate systems for auditing the quality of data are not in place. The UK government is now changing the basis by which hospitals are funded in a way that places a premium on the detailed recording of activity[23]. It will be interesting to see how this affects the quality of clinical coding in hospitals.

Conclusion

The issues that currently surround the creation of patient data seem to be organised around two underlying questions: (1) what is the viability of existing computer-based records as a tool for supporting care; and (2) what further developments are required if such records are to permit the advances that advocates of computerisation were identifying as early as 1966.

A recent review of the relevant research argued that the absence of standardised methods for assessing data quality in patient records means that little can be concluded. 'Accuracy', which might seem a fairly well-defined concept at first sight, has to be translated into something more concrete before it can be measured and can be translated into a variety of different measures. Thiru *et al.* have described a tool kit with a number of measures of both validity and utility. Their research is unusually optimistic about the current state of play in record-keeping in general practice[24].

Perhaps the most interesting study compared paperless to paper-based medical records on a variety of criteria relating to both completeness and legibility[25]. The authors had expected to find that paperless records would be truncated and contain local abbreviations (making them less legible). The reverse was true. Paperless records were more likely to have the diagnosis recorded, contain a record of the advice given and have details of any referral made or treatment prescribed.

The current generation of computer-based records has, it would seem, allowed some improvements over paper-based records. But major difficulties remain. I would set out three goals for an EHR:

• Integration of information across different health care organisations
• The use of routinely collected data as the raw material of medical research
• The development of software that can respond to the content of a patient's history

Achieving clarity of recording and compatibility of systems will involve successful standardisation at several levels. This is why the research is in part about developing terminologies, in part about ontologies and in part about architectures. Of course, even if we get all that right, it will only solve the technical problems.

References

1. Nelson CW. 90th anniversary of the Mayo medical records system. *Mayo Clin Proc* 1997;72(8):696.
2. Swisslog. http://www.swisslog.com/home/references/indu-health/indu-health-case1. htm (accessed on 20 May 2002).
3. Weed LL. Medical records that guide and teach. *N Engl J Med* 1968;278(11): 593–600.
4. Slack WV, Hicks GP, Reed CE, Van Cura LJ. A computer-based medical-history system. *N Engl J Med* 1966;274(4):194–198.
5. Tait I. History of our records. *BMJ* (Clin Res Ed) 1981;282(6265):702–704.
6. Reiser SJ. The clinical record in medicine. Part 2: Reforming content and purpose. *Ann Intern Med* 1991;114(11):980–985.
7. WHO (World Health Organization). *International Statistical Classification of Diseases and Related Health Problems*, 1989 Revision. Geneva: World Health Organization, 1992.
8. NHS Information Authority. *The Clinical Terms Version 3 (The Read Codes)*. Crown Copyright 2000.
9. Snomed International. *Welcome To Snomed*. http://www.snomed.org (accessed on 12 Feb 2004).
10. National Library of Medicine. *Medical Subject Headings*. http://www.nlm.nih.gov/ mesh/meshhome.html (accessed on 12 Feb 2004).

11. Gray J, Orr D, Majeed A. Use of Read Codes in diabetes management in a south London primary care group: implications for establishing disease registers. *BMJ* 2003;326(7399):1130.

12. Gray J, Majeed A, Kerry S, Rowlands G. Identifying patients with ischaemic heart disease in general practice: cross-sectional study of paper and computerised medical records. *BMJ* 2000;321(7260):548–550.

13. Wang SJ, Middleton B, Prosser LA, *et al.* A cost–benefit analysis of electronic medical records in primary care. *Am J Med* 2003;114(5):397–403.

14. Hsia DC, Krushat WM, Fagan AB, Tebbutt JA, Kusserow RP. Accuracy of diagnostic coding for Medicare patients under the prospective-payment system. *N Engl J Med* 1988;318(6):352–355.

15. Van der Lei J. Use and abuse of computer-stored medical records. *Methods Inf Med* 1991;30(2):79–80.

16. Greenhalgh T, Hurwitz B. Narrative based medicine: why study narrative? *BMJ* 1999;318:48–50.

17. Kay S, Purves IN. Medical records and other stories: a narratological framework. *Methods Inf Med* 1996;35(2):72–87.

18. Berg M. Medical work and the computer-based patient record: a sociological perspective. *Methods Inf Med* 1998;37(3):294–301.

19. Tange HJ, Schouten HC, Kester AD, Hasman A. The granularity of medical narratives and its effect on the speed and completeness of information retrieval. *J Am Med Inform Assoc* 1998;5(6):571–582.

20. The OpenEHR Foundation. *OpenEHR.* http://www.openehr.org/ (accessed on 18 July 2003).

21. Bristol Royal Infirmary Inquiry. *Learning from Bristol: The Report of the Public Inquiry into Children's Heart Surgery at the Bristol Royal Infirmary 1984–1995.* London: HMSO, 2001.

22. Audit Commission. *Data Remember.* London: HMSO, 2002.

23. Department of Health. *Reforming NHS Financial Flows: Introducing Payment by Results.* London: Department of Health, 2002.

24. Thiru K, Hassey A, Sullivan F. Systematic review of scope and quality of electronic patient record data in primary care. *BMJ* 2003;326(7398):1070–1075.

25. Hippisley-Cox J, Pringle M, Cater R, *et al.* The electronic patient record in primary care – regression or progression? A cross sectional study. *BMJ* 2003;326:1439–1443.

CHAPTER 3
Creation of medical knowledge

Genomic medicine

On 26 June 2000, Bill Clinton and Tony Blair announced the publication of a usable draft of the human genome, a complete map of human DNA. Media coverage highlighted the enormous potential of genomic science to transform our understanding of disease and to help identify new treatments[1]. There is still much we do not understand about the genome and its role in biological processes: we have not established all the protein-coding sequences in the genome and we know next to nothing about the function of the 98% of the genome that does not code for proteins.* We need to find out more about the pathways and networks by means of which genes and gene products determine the working of cells and larger structures[2]. A particularly significant element of this, which has already been taken up by a major international collaboration (HapMap), is to map the common patterns of heritable variation in the genome[3].

These scientific advances have a quite extraordinary potential to transform practical health care. It is not simply that we will be able to predict a predisposition to those diseases that we know to be genetically determined, although that in itself would be useful for certain conditions. We should be able to establish a new taxonomy for diseases, based on their molecular characterisation. We will develop gene-based approaches to therapeutics and identify the genetic determinants of disease and reactions to drugs.

For example, muscular dystrophies have traditionally been grouped and named according to clinical features, but as our understanding of the genetic and molecular basis for these diseases increases, it may prove more appropriate to classify them according to the physiological mechanisms that underlie the disease[4]. The most common form of inherited lethal musculoskeletal disorder is Duchenne Muscular Dystrophy (DMD), which has an estimated prevalence of 1:3500 live male births. It manifests in early childhood, cripples

---

*We are all familiar with the idea that inheritance works through our genes, that genes are the medium through which our parents give us all the faults they had, and add some extra just for us. DNA also contains the instructions that tell the cells that make up the body how to behave. A particular sequence of DNA is said to 'code' for a protein if it contains instructions that tell a cell how to make that protein. Such proteins are known as gene products.

between the ages of 7 and 12 and kills by the early twenties. It is caused by mutations on the gene Xp21. This is the gene for dystrophin, a protein that interacts with a large protein complex, which is thought to protect muscle fibre membrane from the mechanical stress caused by muscle contraction. DMD is one of a class of diseases now understood to be 'dystrophinopathies'. A significant percentage of patients with these diseases have been found to have mutations known as 'premature stop codons': a metaphorical full stop has been inserted in error into the genetic instructions for the production of dystrophin. An obvious aim for research into the treatment of these patients is therefore to find a way of using products such as gentamicin, which is known to help cells keep reading past such full stops.

Identifying associations between clinical features, protein behaviour and genetic mutations is easiest in the diseases that are 'monogenic', i.e. caused by the behaviour of a single gene. Modes of inheritance have been established for thousands of conditions caused by such mutations in single genes. Most of these diseases, however, are uncommon. Genomics will make a much greater contribution to health care if it proves possible to uncover the mechanisms of common diseases such as diabetes or asthma. We have identified some of the mutations that cause common diseases in some people, e.g. the BRCA1 gene for breast cancer. However, in effect, this means only that we have identified a relatively small subgroup of patients for whom breast cancer is a monogenic disorder. In most cases of common diseases, it will probably be necessary to search for combinations of genes and to identify mutations that are common but which may not always lead to the disease. It will involve looking not just for genes but also for gene–gene interactions and for interactions between genes and other environmental factors[5].

Already our knowledge of the underlying genetics is altering treatment. Researchers looking at a haematology known as diffuse large B-cell lymphoma have used computer algorithms for clustering data to identify a complex genetic signature that allowed the cases they were studying to be classified into two distinct subgroups. This was significant because the two groups had different overall survival rates and demonstrated the possibility of developing individualised treatments based on genetic testing[6].

The potential of these discoveries to revolutionise health care should be obvious. Knowing the genetic basis for a disease and being able to identify those who will prove susceptible to it makes possible to advise on preventative strategies such as changing one's behaviour, undergoing regular screening or prophylactic treatment. In the longer term, understanding the causal chain that goes from genetic mutation, through disruption in the production of proteins to the processes that underlie diseases will help researchers and pharmaceutical companies identify promising starting points for drug development. There are 30 000 protein-coding genes, but as yet only 500 pharmaceuticals that target human gene products.

The sheer scale of data involved in genomic research is mind-boggling, and the field of bioinformatics has grown up to help provide the computational tools required. I want to consider two kinds of study of crucial importance in this research since the techniques they use will be discussed at greater length later on.

Microarray experiments

Proteins are produced from the instructions in a gene by a process known as 'gene expression'. A study often carried out in molecular biology involves establishing a gene expression profile from a sample of DNA. A microarray is a piece of chip technology that measures the extent to which different gene sequences are expressed in a single sample of DNA[7]. The marvel of the technology is that it allows the researcher to test for as many as 100 000 different sequences simultaneously. The result is a rectangular grid, a few centimetres across, holding an array of 100 000 dots roughly 150 μm in diameter; the colour of each dot reflects the extent to which a particular gene, or other DNA sequence, was expressed in the sample. Microarray experiments are expensive and although the amount of data they produce is very large, in terms of the number of sequences tested in each array, the sample size of a study tends to be small. A typical study would attempt to determine whether, in a sample of, say, 40 patients, there was a characteristic pattern of dots for those patients who responded to treatment that was absent for the patients who did not. The mathematical tools that can be used to search for meaningful classifications in the data are similar to those used in other areas of health informatics that deal with similar quantities of data, such as the analysis of medical images.

Cohort studies

In order to identify the contributions made to the risk of disease by genetic factors we also need to carry out a very different kind of experiment, in which large numbers of healthy volunteers are recruited and monitored over many years. The UK Biobank study intends to follow 500 000 people over the coming decades[8]. Each participant will give 50 ml of blood and plasma that will remain available for subsequent analysis. Medical records, including prescription records, will be released and participants will also complete questionnaires providing data about lifestyle, diet and environmental factors. The scale of the study, together with the technology capable of analysing genetic material, will allow many existing hypotheses to be tested in a way that had not previously been possible. The draft protocol lists nine hypotheses, all of which deal with the interplay between specified genetic variants and other factors (cigarette smoking, alcohol consumption, use of hormone therapies, consumption of meat) and their independent and combined impact on the risk of common diseases: ischaemic heart disease, stroke, diabetes, dementia, breast cancer, arthritis. Inevitably it will seem rational to investigate new hypotheses and the design should allow these also to be explored.

Medical knowledge

I want now to look at the specific issue raised in the title of this chapter: the use of patient data to enhance medical knowledge. To understand the scope of health informatics it is important that the concept of medical knowledge be given a broader definition than might be suggested by the above discussion of basic science.

Medical knowledge could be defined as the principles or heuristics that we abstract from experience and use to guide future action. There are various elements to this; most obviously, the current state of scientific knowledge not just in molecular biology but every other relevant discipline from physiology to anatomy and psychotherapy to microsurgery. We would want to include knowledge of different kinds: a basic clinical education in the characteristics of diseases, the varieties of therapeutics and their application. In short, all the sorts of things that we expect health professionals to learn in their academic training.

Medical knowledge could, more broadly, be thought of as encompassing all the things that a health care practitioner needs to know in order to carry out clinical work. This means not just knowing about diseases and diagnoses but also about the organisation of health care and the procedures followed in the institutions through which health care is delivered. Medical knowledge could include such facts as the telephone number that a junior doctor in a particular trust has to call in order to book a computed tomography (CT) scan. This might seem too specific or mundane a fact to be classified as medical knowledge, and we might want to call it information rather than knowledge, but it is worth bearing in mind that readily available accurate and up-to-date information of this sort is essential for the successful treatment of patients and that the poor quality of such 'directory' information is currently a major problem for the NHS and its staff.

This chapter looks at how medical knowledge is created, both in the sense of knowledge about diseases and health problems and the sense of knowledge about how health care organisations operate. There are several processes at work here. Individuals learn from their own experience. Organisations adapt in response to feedback about their performance. Scientific knowledge advances through experiment. The management of health information has some bearing on all these processes. Individual practitioners learn better if they keep clear and accurate records of their decisions and review them once the outcomes are known. Organisations become more efficient and less error-prone if they record data that can be used to audit their performance. Precise and accurate measurements, or other equivalent evaluations, of patient outcomes are the basis on which treatments are compared in scientific studies. The later sections of this chapter set out the ways in which health informatics can be used to aid the processes by which medical knowledge progresses.

Learning from experience

We add to our understanding of what diseases exist, what form they take, how they progress and how they are best treated, by a process that has a number of stages and a number of prerequisites. First, someone has to observe the problem. This might result in the publication of a paper describing an unusual case or series of cases. These papers sometimes seem curiously unscientific to a non-clinical reader. The data presented are not necessarily the results of a trial or an experiment; they are simply the result of observations. The patients described in the paper might represent a subgroup of patients not hitherto studied; they might be victims of a new disease or of a previously unidentified special case of a common complaint.

If the paper is sufficiently interesting, if it either throws down a challenge to those who thought they knew all about an area or if it seems possible that it might affect patient outcomes, it will stimulate new research. This will be, or should be, more obviously experimental in character. The current controversy about the measles, mumps, rubella (MMR) vaccine was stimulated by a paper in the *Lancet* identifying a group of 12 children who all had received the vaccine and had a developmental disorder and an unusual gastrointestinal abnormality[9]. The subsequent furore led to a number of research projects. One group looked at the epidemiological data. They showed, to the satisfaction of most of their colleagues, that although there had been a sharp increase in the diagnosis of autism at the time the MMR vaccine was introduced, the number of children diagnosed with autism had continued to increase steadily while there had been a levelling off of MMR uptake, suggesting that the two were not related[10]. The contrast between this study and the original report could not be starker. The article in the *Lancet* was based on a detailed personal knowledge of a small group of patients, reported by the physician responsible for their care. The subsequent study was based on the analysis of data collected from thousands of patients, known only to the authors through the fragments extracted from their medical records. A third group undertook another form of investigation, using molecular techniques to ascertain that measles virus genomes were present in patients who had both the developmental disorder and the gastrointestinal abnormality but were not present in a series of controls[11].

Research paradigms

The term 'paradigm' is often used to denote a particular approach to research. Research paradigms vary, for example, in the extent to which they deal with quantitative or qualitative data, whether they are objective or subjective, or experimental as opposed to observational. Let us look at these three distinctions more closely.

We say that a research study is quantitative if the data generated by the study are numerical. It does not matter what is being counted or measured – it might be the patient's temperature, the proportion of cancer cases correctly identified by the doctor, the mean waiting time of outpatients or the number of nurses who rated a system as satisfactory. So long as the outcome is expressed as a quantity, the research is quantitative. Qualitative research, which can be just as rigorous, generates different kinds of data. One common technique is the methodical analysis of interview transcripts to identify significant themes. Such research is extremely valuable in assessing the attitudes or reactions of patients and practitioners. (See Box 3.1 for an example of a system using qualitative data.)

Most researchers attempt to be objective, to report their observations free from the taint of their own expectations or prejudices. Most of us generally accept, perhaps without thinking too much about it, that there is such a thing as ultimate truth and that the job of science is to discover as much of it as possible. There is, however, a contrary view, which holds that all observations are inherently subjective and those that scientists attempt to pass off as the truth, or as an approximation of it, are merely views with no more claim to authority than any other. On this view, research that acknowledges its subjectivity is more honest and perhaps more valuable. This view is much more common in the social than the physical sciences. One example of a subjectivist paradigm is 'participatory' research, in which the researchers actively engage with the organisation or setting they seek to study. In 'action research', for example, researchers may work with members of an organisation and help them understand and improve its operation.

The final distinction is between experimental and observational research. There is a view of science, sometimes called Popperian after the philosopher Karl Popper, which holds that the aim of experiments is to attempt to prove hypotheses false. The scientific method, then, involves first forming a theory or conjecture and then testing it through experiment. Not all research follows this pattern, however. Some researchers publish purely descriptive findings, not the results of an experiment or attempts to test a theory, but simply an account of what was observed.

Different paradigms will give different kinds of answers and therefore tend to be applied to different kinds of questions. Research that takes a subjectivist stance, uses observational methods and deals in qualitative data is more commonly used in those areas of medical research that shade into sociology or psychology. Research that sets out to be objective, experimental and quantitative is usually grounded in the physical sciences. There is not a straightforward dichotomy here, however. How would one classify an economic evaluation of lung cancer screening, a comparison of patients' attitudes to telephone versus face-to-face consultations or an attempt to measure the impact of acupuncture on back pain? Research can be subjective and also quantitative or experimental but still qualitative.

The rest of this chapter looks in detail at three different ways in which patient data can be used: case studies, longitudinal surveys and clinical trials.

Box 3.1 Database of individual patient experiences (DIPEX)

Most medical research is concerned, at some level, with measurement. Different medical sciences measure different things. Some measure attributes of individual cells, others look at the behaviour of whole organs, while still others are interested in how people, groups and indeed whole populations can be assessed on some measure or set of measures. The unit of study and the method will vary but by and large there is something that is being quantified. Much that is of interest to us, however, is hard to quantify, and some researchers, who are more concerned with understanding the nature of the experience of illness, work in a different paradigm, using what are known as qualitative (as opposed to quantitative) methods.

One interesting project in health informatics, DIPEX (www.dipex.org), aims to provide recently diagnosed patients with an understanding of what they are likely to experience as they go through their treatment and learn to live with its effects. The idea is to elicit information from patients who have already been through the experience, analyse the resulting data – which are essentially interview transcripts – and present the results on a website in a way that combines the psychological force of personal testimony with the greater reliability of evidence gathered from a cross section of patients.

The website provides an interesting contrast to others described in this book, e.g. the PubMed website of the National Institute of Health in the USA. Such sites hope to have an impact through the improved decision-making that will result from doctors, and in some cases patients, having better access to more accurate information about diseases and treatments. DIPEX is different. It is not primarily aimed at influencing decisions. Rather the hope is that patients will be better able to cope with frightening diagnoses or traumatic treatments having seen or heard what other patients said about similar experiences.

The 'experiences' section of the website, which also includes a discussion forum, is organised around a set of modules, defined around broad – mainly diagnostic – categories such as breast cancer, heart failure or epilepsy. The information in each module is indexed thematically and by patient. The user can either review biographical information about the patient, perhaps to find someone in similar circumstances to themselves, or may search the thematic index for an extract that deals with a particular issue.

The modules are built up from interviews. The interviewees are not a random sample of patients with the condition. Rather the sample is put together, following consultation with experts and patients, to guarantee coverage of the relevant issues. Unlike most quantitative studies where the sample size is determined in advance, the strategy is to keep adding to the sample until the full range of patient experiences is covered. Most modules are based on 40–50 interviews. The researchers, who generally have a background in the social sciences, interview patients, usually in their own homes. The interviews are taped, sometimes videotaped, and the tapes are then transcribed and analysed. The analysis involves dividing the interview into segments, associating each segment with a topic and then identifying significant topics.

The set of significant topics is used to provide the thematic links between the different patient interviews. The researchers then draft 'topic summaries' that bring together segments addressing the key topics. The final step in the creation of the module involves selecting audio and video clips to illustrate the key points that emerge from the interviews.

The result is a site, which, by virtue of the careful approach to sampling, interview and analysis, can hope to provide information and support on the most significant questions that emerge from patients' experience of diagnosis, treatment and living with the consequences of illness. Unlike many other sites, the information is presented from the patient's perspective in terms that patients will recognise and understand.

Case studies

In September 1994 doctors at Guy's Hospital in London examined a 16-year-old girl of Cypriot origin[12]. She had been injured in a fall the previous March and subsequently developed backache and numbness in her face and fingers. By August her speech was slurred, her balance poor and she was becoming clumsier. The doctors observed poor recall and dyscalculia. Her condition continued to deteriorate and she died soon afterwards. A biopsy of the frontal lobe revealed spongiform changes and plaques.

Around the same time doctors in Bristol were treating an 18-year-old man who had been referred for depression[13]. His memory was deteriorating and he suffered from hallucinations and delusions as well as a fear of water and sharp objects, which meant he had stopped washing or shaving. His parents observed that he had become apathetic and confused, unable to carry out simple tasks like unlocking a door or boiling an egg. His doctors described him as somnolent, ataxic and dysathric. He was admitted to residential care where staff noted that he would sometimes scream without there being an obvious source of alarm. Less than a year after the onset of his illness he was dead. Biospy again revealed evidence of spongiform change.

Both these cases were histopathologically confirmed as Creutzfeldt–Jakob disease (CJD), an illness rare in the population as a whole but vanishingly rare in young people. In both cases the doctors were sufficiently surprised at this to write letters for publication in the *Lancet*, describing the case and giving details of their diagnosis. A year after the publication of these letters, the *Lancet* published a paper announcing the identification of what was, in effect, a new disease: new variant CJD or nvCJD[14]. By then ten cases had been identified and a distinctive neuropathological profile described.

The detailed description of an individual case is generally considered useful either because it is typical of the disease or because it is not. Typical cases are especially important in education; if we use good examples our explanations of categories are clearer. They also serve a role in research: if one is going to study an example in detail, one should use a good example. But we are also intrigued by unusual cases that can serve to modify or extend our idea of an existing concept, such as a disease. Cases are sometimes highlighted because they cannot be understood in terms of any existing classification: they demand a more profound rethink, such as the identification of a new disease.

Consider the problem from a statistical perspective. Let each case be described by a set of terms. Let us give each term a number. Imagine, for simplicity's sake, that each number represents the value of some important clinical parameter: e.g. temperature or pulse rate. If each parameter is given a dimension, the set of numbers can be used as a set of coordinates, to allocate the case to a point in some n-dimensional space. We can let n be 2; it will be less plausible clinically, but easier to draw. The classification of cases is, mathematically, a matter of defining distinct regions of space within which clusters of cases that can be considered together, perhaps because they are susceptible to a common clinical approach, are found (see Figure 3.1). Clinical categories are sometimes defined by precise ranges of numeric values (hypertension in terms of blood pressure, diabetes in terms of blood sugar), but more commonly through a set of characteristics not all of which will be present in every case. Imagine a region of space that is defined by a central 'typical' case. Other cases are classified not by the measurement of any individual dimension but according to their distance from the typical case.

A new case might show that the boundaries of the region were drawn too tightly. Or a sequence of new cases might show that the model is wrong in a more fundamental sense. Perhaps we were considering as one disease a set of cases that would be better understood as two or more diseases. Perhaps the way we have constructed our space is inaccurate, and a useful classification will require hitherto unrecognised dimensions. For example, there is a known association between cholesterol and heart disease. There is a causal link because cholesterol can lead to atherosclerosis, deposits of atheroma plaque in the walls of arteries. One could plot total cholesterol levels against incidence of coronary heart disease and find a correlation. There is, however, a stronger association between cholesterol and heart disease that is to do with the relative concentrations of two forms of carrier molecule, used to transport cholesterol through the blood stream. Low-density lipoprotein particles take cholesterol onto the sites where the body makes use of it, high-density ones take it back to the liver for excretion. A patient with a high measurement of total cholesterol may be at less risk than a patient in whom a lower total measurement contains a disproportionately high

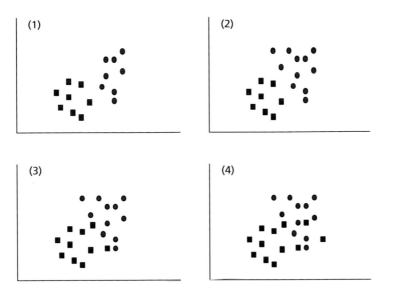

Figure 3.1 A set of clinical cases classified on two dimensions. Let the squares be cases we would classify as disease A and the circles cases we would classify as disease B. Looking at the data in the first plot, it seems as though we can use the property measured on the x-axis to distinguish between the two diseases. In the second plot, new data mean that this is no longer the case, but the two sets are still clearly separable. The data added in the third plot make the separation less clear. We have cases on the line that would separate the two. In the fourth plot, it is plain that the diseases cannot be distinguished on these two dimensions.

concentration of low-density lipoprotein particles. We need to consider not the single dimension of total cholesterol but the two dimensions of high-density and low-density lipoprotein concentration.

The refinement and reorganisation of classifications is a fundamental part of the process by which knowledge advances. In cancer, for example, the treatment given will depend on the 'stage' of the cancer. Staging criteria are periodically refined or revised. The more closely we study the effectiveness of treatments, the more accurate our classification can be. Other factors also come into play: we may wish to classify patients not just by disease or stage but according to whether in any given case a disease has a genetic cause, and then to specify the gene.

The microarray experiments used in the study of diffuse large B-cell lymphoma that were mentioned in the start of this chapter employed computer algorithms to derive a classification of DNA samples, which proved to correlate with the effectiveness of treatment. The data consisted of a small number of samples, where the samples conceptually had many dimensions. The goal of the classification was not to separate out the different dots in each microarray but to separate out two different groups of patients on the basis of the measurements given in the microarray. In terms of the graphs presented above, the graph for a typical microarray study would have a pretty similar number of points on it but would have 100 000 dimensions rather than just 2.

To return to the example at the start of this section, it would be simplistic to suggest that nvCJD was identified purely because of the case reports published in the *Lancet*. There was already public concern about the possibility that one could catch a spongiform disease from eating beef infected with bovine spongiform encephalopathy (BSE) that had led to the setting up of a unit to monitor incidence of CJD. In that sense the case reports were not so much a challenge to existing thinking about CJD as a novel but not unexpected development. This is an important point. In real life, data very often do not fit exactly into the expected categories and so unexpected results are, in general, not all that unexpected. They succeed in changing our view of the world only if they show us a new way of looking at things that is either more consistent with a range of troubling results or has some other intuitive appeal.

If there had not been talk about the threat of a human version of BSE, would the cases have been diagnosed as CJD? And even if they had, would the clinicians have thought it worthwhile to report a rare but not unheard-of event (CJD in a young person had been reported before, though not in the UK), and if they had not how long would it have been before someone collated the statistics from different parts of the country and identified the dramatic increase in incidence?

Improved health information management should allow the collation of accurate disease registers that will help researchers to monitor more effectively the incidence of disease and to improve our understanding of the genetic and environmental factors that affect health. These kinds of epidemiological study are another way in which patient data is used to generate medical knowledge.

Longitudinal surveys

Framingham is a prosperous community 20 miles west of Boston. It is the largest town in Massachusetts and the home of the first man to die in the War of Independence. Since 1948 it has also been the subject of an extraordinary exercise in the collection and analysis of patient data[15]. Researchers seeking to understand the causes of cardiovascular disease recruited 5209 men and women between the ages of 30 and 62 who, every 2 years, return for interviews, physical examinations and laboratory tests. Within 4 years, 34 heart attacks had been recorded and high blood pressure, high blood cholesterol and obesity had been identified as possible risk factors. As the years have passed, the investigators have been able to study a greater range of factors and to explore how they relate, using increasingly sophisticated measurement and imaging technology. In recent years the focus has been on the identification of the genetic component of cardiovascular disease. Since 1971, 5124 of the original participants' children have been recruited into a second study and it is now hoped to recruit 3500 of the original cohort's grandchildren. This is the kind of prospective longitudinal study that the UK Biobank, mentioned above, seeks to emulate.

The data provided by the Framingham study have proved exceptionally useful. By following a population of this size, monitoring physiological indices and lifestyle factors and examining their relationship with the incidence of heart disease, researchers have been able to identify, and quantify, the major risk factors: high blood pressure, high total cholesterol with high-density lipoprotein concentration, smoking, obesity, diabetes and physical inactivity.

The mathematics behind this analysis is based on a technique called regression. Let us again consider a problem that can be represented in two dimensions. Imagine that we know the heights and weights of a group of people and we want to predict the weight of another person whose height we know. We can plot the heights and weights that we know and draw the straight line that represents the best fit with the data. Once we have this line, we can work out a predicted weight for any given height. How good the prediction is depends on two things: the extent to which our data is a good sample of the relevant population, and the strength of the underlying relationship – the correlation – between height and weight. The mathematics is pretty simple. The general equation for a straight line is

$$y = a + bx$$

So once you know the line, you have values for a and b and can obtain a value for y for any given x. The same mathematics can be used for multivariate regression, where the variable to be predicted depends on more than one input variable, so the equation is

$$y = a + b_1x_1 + b_2x_2 + b_3x_3 + b_4x_4 + b_nx_n$$

In cases such as the prediction of cardiovascular risk, many 'predictor' variables are not numeric quantities but observations that are either true or false. In such cases we represent true as 1 and false as 0. Risk is numeric, but can take values only in a certain range (limited at one end by impossibility and at the other by certainty). The mathematics of regression require that we transform these quantities into something that is linear, compute the regression, then transform them back. The transformation, known as logit, replaces a value x by $\ln(x/1 - x)$ so that the equation for what is called logistic regression is

$$\ln(p/1 - p) = a + b_1x_1 + b_2x_2 + b_3x_3 + b_4x_4 + b_nx_n$$

where p is, for example, the 10-year risk of cardiovascular disease.

The Framingham researchers have used their regression equations to generate tables that allow you to calculate the 10-year risk of cardiovascular disease for a given set of risk factors. A 37-year-old man with a systolic blood pressure of 140 mmHg and total cholesterol of 170 mg/dl and high-density lipoprotein concentration of 55 mg/dl and who is not diabetic has a 4%

chance of developing coronary heart disease by the age of 47, if he does not smoke[16]. The risk almost doubles if he smokes. These equations have become extremely well known and have been made the basis for graphical tools to help predict risk. Numerous websites also use the equations in online calculators, again to predict risk. Such tools are used by the general public, motivated by anxiety or curiosity, but also by GPs who increasingly believe that it does not make sense to manage, for example, hypertension (high blood pressure) in isolation, and that decisions about treatment should follow an assessment of a patient's overall risk[17].

The contrast between the success of the Framingham equations and the failure of the AAPHelp system, described in Chapter 1, is instructive. Both projects used mathematical tools that would be unfamiliar to most clinicians to derive numeric estimates of the risk of disease in a particular patient. Clinicians have been happy to adopt the Framingham risk-factor model and use the mathematical tools in dealing with their patients. The significant difference between this and the AAPHelp system is in the data collection. Remember that de Dombal concluded that 'databases don't travel'. The Framingham risk equations have been applied in different settings and among different populations. In the AAPHelp system the data were collected simply to support the implementation of a system; this ended up constraining the system by localizing it to a setting in which data were collected. The Framingham study was designed as an epidemiological survey, so the data were collected from a more broadly representative sample, which allowed the findings to be treated as generalisable medical knowledge, established through research. This was only later built into software calculators. The notion of the 'risk factor', invented by the Framingham investigators, has entered the clinical vocabulary. The identified risk factors, and indeed the equations based on them, have proved more robust than the Bayesian probabilities studied by the AAPHelp team. Clinicians using the Framingham equations may not feel that they have grasped the mathematics behind the model or that they could do the calculations themselves but they do feel that they understand the medical basis for the predictions in a way that the users of AAPHelp probably did not.

Increasingly, medical research is generating knowledge about risk. Surveys like the Framingham study have identified risk factors for a range of diseases. Known risk factors for breast cancer include the number of first-degree relatives with the disease, age, use of hormone replacement therapy (HRT), smoking, social class and age at first childbirth. Studies of other diseases have uncovered links with diet, exercise, contraceptive use and so on. As our understanding of the genetic basis of certain diseases increases, we will be more able to identify who is at risk from which diseases and how great these risks are. One of the most important tasks for health informatics in the coming years is to develop the tools that will enable this information to be used to best effect. We need tools that help doctors calculate the prior probability of a patient having a disease before they recommend a test. We need tools to help patients decide how best to weigh up the risks and benefits of the various options open to them.

Randomised controlled trials

After Britain joined the War of the Austrian Succession in 1740, Commodore Anson led a squadron of six ships, which left England with the object of rounding Cape Horn and attacking Spanish colonies on the Pacific coast. He finally returned, almost 4 years later, having circumnavigated the globe, captured a Spanish galleon of immense value in the Philippines and seen action off the coasts of Chile and Peru. Perhaps the most extraordinary fact about the voyage, however, is that, of the 1955 men who set out, 997 had died of scurvy by the time Anson returned to England. In 1753 James Lind, a Scottish naval surgeon, published a *Treatise on the Scurvy*, dedicated to Anson, by then Admiral of the Fleet[18]. In it he describes the following experiment:

> On the 20th of May 1747; I took twelve patients in the scurvy, on board the *Salisbury* at sea. Their cases were as similar as I could have them. They all in general had putrid gums, the spots and lassitude, with weakness of the knees. They lay together in one place being a proper apartment for the sick in the fore-hold; and had one diet in common to all.... Two of them were ordered each a quart of cider a day. Two others took twenty-five gutts of elixir vitriol three times a day upon an empty stomach; using a gargle strongly acidulated with it for their mouths. Two others took two spoonfuls of vinegar three times a day, upon an empty stomach; having their gruels and other foods well acidulated with it, as also the gargle for their mouth. Two of the worst patients with the tendons in the right ham rigid (a symptom none of the rest had) were put under a course of seawater. Of this they drank half a pint every day, and sometimes more or less as it operated, by way of gentle physic. Two others had each two oranges and one lemon given them every day. These they ate with greediness, at different times, upon an empty stomach. They continued but six days under this course having consumed the quantity that could be spared. The two remaining patients took the bigness of a nutmeg three times a day of an electuary recommended by an hospital surgeon...
>
> The consequence was that the most sudden and visible good effects were perceived from the use of oranges and lemons; one of those who had taken them being at the end of six days fit for duty.... The other was the best recovered of any in his condition; and being now deemed pretty well, was appointed nurse to the rest of the sick.

This experiment was probably the world's first 'randomised controlled trial' (RCT). Such experiments are now regarded as providing the best and most secure foundation for ascertaining the effectiveness of treatments. It is possible to discover whether or not a treatment works only by means of experiments on real patients: the treatment must be given to a group of patients and data then collected about the consequences for those patients' outcomes. Such experiments are called clinical trials. In order to allow a fair assessment of the effects of any treatment, data must also be collected describing what happens, or what happened, in the absence of that treatment. If such data are collected, we say that the study is 'controlled'. Ideally, we want to compare what happens when the treatment is given (the intervention condition) with what happens when it is not given (the control condition) in the knowledge that the only difference between the two groups is whether or not they receive the treatment. To be certain of this, the best thing to do is randomly to assign patients (or consultations, or doctors, or hospitals or whatever the unit of study is) to either the intervention or the control condition. RCTs provide the most secure basis on which valid causal inferences can be made about the effects of medical interventions.

From Lind's account it seems that patients were assigned randomly to the different conditions – although now we would expect to be given details of the randomisation process. We are assured that their cases were as similar as possible. We are also told that, in terms of where they were cared for and of their general diet, they were managed in the same way. The intervention (citrus fruits) is compared with a number of controls, including the contemporary recommendation of best practice. The outcomes are reported clearly, and seem to show a significant difference in favour of the intervention. There were only two patients in each condition so the sample size is obviously small, and one could also question the length of follow-up. Nevertheless, it meets enough of our criteria to be described as a valid RCT.

In order to understand the role of the RCT in medicine it is important to understand its limitations. The RCT essentially poses a single question: it has a binary outcome, a yes or no answer. This means that it is not an effective instrument for many kinds of investigation: there are areas where our ignorance is such that we are not in a position to formulate the sorts of questions that can be answered in an RCT. It is, however, the most effective instrument for answering questions about the relative effectiveness of two treatments or about the effectiveness of a treatment compared to no treatment or to a placebo.

Say we have enrolled 100 patients for a trial of a new drug. Of these, 50 patients are randomly assigned to receive the drug currently given (the control group); 50 receive the new drug (the intervention group). Ideally we would want neither the patients nor their doctors to know whether they were in the intervention or control groups; if this were possible, we would say that the trial was double-blinded. Clearly it is easier to do this if two drugs are being compared than if the trial is assessing the value of amputation. Let us stick with drugs. What could be concluded if 30 of the 50 patients in the control group responded, compared to 35 of the patients in the intervention group. The difference between the two proportions is $35/50 - 30/50 = 0.1$. Is this difference big enough to show that the new drug is better? Might it not just be a matter of chance? The mathematics of 'sampling distributions' allows us to compute a measure of the statistical variation that can be expected for samples drawn at random from a set. The same mathematics can be used to calculate the expected variation of a difference between two proportions. It turns out that, assuming our 100 patients are representative of the wider population of interest, we can estimate that in 95% of samples the difference in proportions would fall in the range −0.08 to +0.28. (See Chapter 11 for a more detailed account of this kind of statistical thinking.) Since this range includes zero, we cannot be 95% confident that the real difference between the two proportions is not zero. So our experiment, like many others, has not shown that the new drug was more effective than conventional treatment.

The 'confidence interval' above was obtained by feeding the numbers from the study − 35/50 and 30/50 − into the equations describing variation in sampling distributions. The calculation of confidence, therefore, is nothing to do with clinical realities, the life stories of patients or the professional qualities of a research team. It simply reflects the brute fact that samples of 50 are on the small side for assessing a difference in proportions, so only a larger effect than in this example would allow anything to be inferred with the degree of confidence that clinical science conventionally requires.

One UK website contains records of more than 15 000 RCTs taking place at the moment[19]. Pharmaceutical companies, universities, charities and other organisations are all involved in evermore complex and intricate trials addressing increasingly detailed questions about treatments. The design, management and analysis of these trials is now a huge business. The regulatory framework for such work has also grown more stringent; a researcher must not just secure funding for the trial but also obtain ethical approval from the institutions responsible for the patient's care, demonstrate that the mechanisms proposed for the collection and analysis of data protect the patients' right to confidentiality and, last but not least, obtain informed consent from all of the participating patients.

Many trials fail because they are unable to recruit an adequate number of patients. Conversely, many patients who would benefit from the early access to treatment and careful monitoring that trials involve are never alerted to the existence of a relevant trial by their physicians.

There is a great deal of work to be done in improving the design, management and analysis of trials. Health informatics can be useful: computer software can help in the design of trials; web-based databases of clinical trials can improve recruitment, alerting clinicians to the existence of trials; purpose-built tools intended to manage the data collection and analysis enable the secure management of complex trials.

Conclusion

Lind's experiment did not bring about an immediate revolution in the management of scurvy. The general use of lemon juice was not mandated throughout the navy until 1793[20]. Within 2 years scurvy had all but disappeared. Why were Lind's results not accepted sooner? There are a number of possible reasons. It was only a small trial and only one of the patients completely recovered. The limitations of the experiment were not probably very significant; it is more that clinical practice takes time to change in response to evidence of any sort.

Careful observation allows valuable lessons to be learnt about the effectiveness of treatments, often, as was the case with Lind, in the absence of any understanding of the explanation. Experiment plays a role, but a single dramatic result is rarely sufficient to overturn a consensus or to change established patterns of thought and behaviour. Medical knowledge today is thoroughly grounded in scientific practice, and medical research is expected to proceed by experiment. It would, however, be extremely Whiggish to assume that we have, through gradual intellectual progress, arrived at a peak of scientific rationality even assuming that we want medicine to be scientific and rational. It currently takes around 6 years to go from thinking of a research question, to securing funding and approval, to recruitment and analysis and finally to completion and publication of a clinical trial. Once the results are published it can still take a number of years before sufficient supporting evidence is gathered for the results to be considered conclusive. Even then there is often a further delay before a new treatment becomes standard practice. Chapter 4 considers how health informatics can help improve clinicians' access to up-to-date clinical evidence.

References

1. BBC. Scientists crack human code. http://news.bbc.co.uk/1/hi/sci/tech/805803.stm
2. Collins FS, Green ED, Guttmacher AE, Guyer MS. A vision for the future of genomics research. *Nature* 2003;422(6934):835–847.
3. The International HapMap Consortium. The International HapMap Project. *Nature* 2003;426(6968):789–796.
4. Wagner KR. Genetic diseases of muscle. *Neurol Clin N Am* 2002;20:648–678.
5. Guttmacher AE, Collins FS. Genomic medicine: a primer. *N Engl J Med* 2002;347:1512–1520.
6. Golub TR. Genomic approaches to the pathogenesis of hematologic malignancy. *Curr Opin Hematol* 2001;81:252–261.
7. Lesk AM. *Introduction to Bioinformatics*. Oxford: Oxford University Press, 2002.
8. UK Biobank. Welcome to the UK BioBank. www.ukbiobank.ac.uk
9. Wakefield AJ, Murch SH, Anthony A, *et al.* Ileal-lymphoid-nodular hyperplasia, non-specific colitis, and pervasive developmental disorder in children. *Lancet* 1998;351(9103):637–641.
10. Taylor B, Miller E, Lingam R, *et al.* Measles, mumps, and rubella vaccination and bowel problems or developmental regression in children with autism: population study. *BMJ* 2002;324(7334):393–396.
11. Uhlmann V, Martin CM, Sheils O, *et al.* Potential viral pathogenic mechanism for new variant inflammatory bowel disease. *Mol Pathol* 2002;55(2):84–90.

12. Britton TC, Al-Serraj S, Shaw C, Campbell T, Collinge J. Sporadic Creutzfeldt–Jakob disease in a 16-year-old in the UK. *Lancet* 1995;346:1155.
13. Bateman D, Hitton D, Love S, Zeidler M, Beck J, Collinge J. Sporadic Creutzfeldt–Jakob disease in an 18-year-old in the UK. *Lancet* 1995;346:1155–1156.
14. Will RG, Ironside J, Zeidler M, *et al.* A new variant of Creutzfeldt–Jakob disease in the UK. *Lancet* 1996;347:921–925.
15. National Heart Lung and Blood Institute. The Framingham Heart Study. http://www.nhlbi.nih.gov/about/framingham/index.html
16. National Cholesterol Education Program. Risk assessment tool for estimating 10-year risk of developing hard CHD (myocardial infarction and coronary death). http://hin.nhlbi.nih.gov/atpiii/calculator.asp?usertype=prof
17. Jackson R, Lawes CM, Bennett DA, Milne RJ, Rodgers A. Treatment with drugs to lower blood pressure and blood cholesterol based on an individual's absolute cardiovascular risk. *Lancet* 2005;365(9457):434–441.
18. Lind J. *A Treatise of the Scurvy in Three Parts*. London, A. Millar, 1753. Available online at: http://www.jameslindlibrary.org/trial_records/17th_18th_Century/lind/lind_kp.html (accessed on 18 July 2003)
19. Current Controlled Trials. Welcome to current controlled trials. http://www.controlled-trials.com/ (accessed on 18 July 2003)
20. Porter R. *The Greatest Benefit to Mankind*. London: Fontana Press, 1999.

CHAPTER 4
Access to medical knowledge

The story of Isabel Maude

Chickenpox, or varicella, is usually a trivial disease, a minor event of child-hood. Some children, however, develop severe skin infections along with chickenpox, and some of these can have serious consequences. In April 1999, three-year-old Isabel Maude fell victim to toxic shock and necrotising fasciitis 4 days after contracting chickenpox[1]. She went on to suffer multiple organ failure including cardiac arrest and was on life support in a paediatric inten-sive care unit (ICU) for nearly 4 weeks and spent 1 month after that in hospital. Her life was in extreme danger and there was a strong possibility of brain damage. In the days before she was admitted to hospital, her parents had been sufficiently worried to consult their GP and their local A&E depart-ment. The medical staff they saw failed to recognise the complications of chickenpox from which Isabel was suffering. And yet these complications, although unusual, are documented.

I am writing this chapter on a networked personal computer. The clock says 10.32 am. I start up a Web browser, go to the PubMed website (the National Institute of Medicine's online database of published medical re-search), type in *varicella* and *fasciitis* as search terms. This simple search finds 32 articles, mainly in paediatric and dermatological journals, but there is also one from the *BMJ*. It turns out to be a comment on a 1996 article, again from the *BMJ*. Ironically this article is by the team at St Mary's Hospital Paddington, the hospital where Isabel Maude was treated. I can access the electronic version of the *BMJ* via a link from PubMed. Another mouse click and I have the full text in front of me. The article seems very clear and accessible, and the third sentence of the first paragraph refers to a recent increase in reports of serious bacterial infections, both during and after chickenpox[2]. The clock says 10.34 am. The whole process has taken less than 2 min. If this information is easy to find, why could it not have been found by the doctors who first saw Isabel?

There are three reasons. First, rather obviously, I am working in an office with a networked PC. A junior doctor in a busy clinic is under different pressures and does not have such easy access to the relevant databases. Second, I knew what I was looking for when I started my literature search. If I had tried to search PubMed using a list of symptoms I would have got nowhere. The third reason is more subtle. How do doctors and other health care workers recognise when there is something that they do not know? Or when something they have learnt is out of date? Behind these three considerations lie problems that come close to defining the field of health informatics. How can we build systems that quickly provide accurate information to busy people working in chaotic places? How can we help people find answers to poorly defined questions? How can we provide alarms and reminders that alert decision-makers to possible problems?

Doctors' use of information sources

For the paediatric intensive care doctors who treated Isabel the underlying problem is familiar. The knowledge required to deal with conditions like Isabel's exists in the health system but in too many cases it is not available to the front-line staff most likely to have the opportunity to make an early diagnosis. The evidence for this is more than anecdotal. Ely *et al.* carried out a study on the information requirements of family doctors[3]. The researchers waited in the corridor during consultations and then, in between consultations, spoke briefly to the doctors to identify the questions that had arisen. The researchers were not interested in the kinds of questions that can be answered by looking at the record, but rather in questions about medical knowledge: 'what is the name of this kind of rash?' or 'what is the right dose for this drug?'. The doctors generated 1101 questions during the study, an average of 0.32 questions per patient. Of these, 702 (64%) were not pursued. Doctors said that they might at a later date seek answers to 123 of these questions. For a further 148 they said that on reflection they were confident that they knew enough to take the right decision. Which leaves 431 questions that were never going to be answered.

Most (80%) of the 399 questions that were pursued were answered. Most of the solutions ($n = 291$, 92%) directly answered the question posed, whereas 27 (8%) provided information related to the question. The answers came from 156 different sources. One of the most revealing findings of the study was that the mean time spent pursuing an answer was 118 s and the median time was 60 s. Unless the answer can be found in less than 2 min, the question will simply never be pursued.

In a similar study, Covell *et al.* monitored 47 generalists and specialists practising internal medicine in 'office practice'[4]. They found that 269 questions came up in 409 patient visits, roughly 2 questions for every 3 patients seen. Only one-third of these questions were answered. Covell *et al.* concluded that 'in a typical half-day of office practice, four management decisions might have been altered if needed information was available at the time of the patient visit'.

This chapter deals with how doctors – and other staff – who are most directly concerned with patient care can be provided with easy and convenient access to the ever-expanding corpus of medical knowledge. The story of Isabel Maude is of interest, not just as a reminder of how serious the consequences of clinical ignorance can be but also because her experience inspired her parents and her doctors to set up a medical charity, with the aim of providing a software solution to this problem. Others have tried to use computers to provide rapid access to relevant information for front-line clinicians, but their approach is distinctive and interesting. Before considering these approaches, however, we should review some of the more conventional solutions. First, we will look at the three most obvious, and most traditional, sources of clinical information: colleagues, books and journals. Each of these has advantages and disadvantages and changes in how new technology allows us to access them.

Colleagues

In 36% of the cases in which the doctors in the Ely *et al.* study did attempt to answer a question, they did so by contacting a colleague. This is the easiest, most familiar and most common route to additional information or specialist knowledge. There are clear advantages to it. It fulfils a social purpose as well as an information-gathering role. A phone call is quick and convenient and having a conversation about a problem allows us to elaborate our thinking about a problem and makes it more likely that we will get the right answer. Human beings are alert to the social and clinical context in which questions arise and more likely than computers to suggest relevant information. But there are problems with relying on colleagues to answer questions.

First, and perhaps most obviously, there is a risk that the person being asked the question will be no better placed to answer it than the person who asked it. In such circumstances a false sense of reassurance may be generated by a colleague who is equally uninformed. A more subtle point is made by Weinberg *et al.*[5] They asked 69 physicians who they turned to for advice about heart disease and found that 90% of queries were dealt with by a core group of six physicians. Informal communication networks can generate enormous inefficiencies. From the point of view of the doctor asking the question, it may seem just a quick phone call; from the point of view of the person being rung, frequent interruptions may be an unwelcome and even stressful distraction.

It is also worth noting that although talking to colleagues may be an enjoyable and even psychologically necessary element in a working day, the pressures generated by social interaction can create problems. Asking a question involves admitting ignorance, which is acceptable if the question is outside one's speciality or if one is talking to somebody one knows and trusts, but may not be otherwise. Equally a clinician may feel that he or she should not be seen to ask too many questions, or may not want to ask the same question twice.

Electronic access to colleagues

Some of the problems associated with the traditional ways of soliciting information from colleagues can be addressed by using different forms of communications technology. Someone wishing to contact a colleague can now choose to telephone his or her desk number, mobile number, send a text, leave a voice message, send an email or use a pager. Much has been written about the impact of email and mobile telephones on modern life. In clinical fields most of the discussion has concerned the use of these forms of technology to support communication with patients, but relatively little has been said about how they can improve communications between professionals.

Sending an email is a simple alternative to making a telephone call and one that allows the recipient to answer the question at his or her convenience. Hospitals are known to be stressful environments in which to work and this is in part because members of staff are frequently interrupted with requests of various kinds. If a significant volume of communication can be shifted from a synchronous (interrupt) mode to an asynchronous mode (such as email), the overall efficiency of the organisation should improve[6].

Two other forms of electronic communication between colleagues are worth mentioning: communities of practice and telemedicine. There are a variety of online discussion groups, news groups and bulletin boards for the exclusive use of clinicians. Some function as mutual support networks. Others, in which people seek to deepen their knowledge and experience in a field, are termed online 'communities of practice'[7]. These online communities are defined, in part, through a shared purpose, interest or need, which very often is the exchange of information. A good example would be the mailing list set up in 1994 to discuss the holistic care of ICU patients; another was set up for psychiatric nurse researchers[8,9]. Such groups have advantages and disadvantages as sources of information. It is easy and acceptable to ask questions, including questions that one might be reluctant to ask a colleague face to face. A much wider body of experience and opinion is potentially available to provide an answer, but it is inevitably harder to know how to assess the significance of the response.

In the course of the 1980s and 1990s researchers interested in how the new forms of communications technology could alter the practice of medicine began to use the term telemedicine for various applications that allowed geographical and organisational boundaries to be breached[10]. Many of these applications involved videoconferencing technology and most were aimed at allowing patients access to remote physicians. Some of the applications, however, involved communication between professionals. The technology has, many people now feel, failed to transfer from research to routine use except where the distances involved make face-to-face consultations impractical[11]. It is difficult to say exactly why it failed and the reasons probably vary from application to application. Many professionals were surprised by the ways in which the technology disturbed their normal routine practice and found it hard to adapt[12]. One area of telemedicine that does seem to have been successful is teleradiology, which allows a radiologist to interpret a digital image (and medical images are increasingly created with digital equipment) sent over a network, or even the Internet[13]. This makes it a great deal easier to seek a second opinion on an image or to send a case to a distant specialist for immediate attention.

Books

Another common place to look for knowledge and information to help answer a clinical question is the textbook. The advantages of textbooks should be obvious enough. They are accessible, portable, familiar and authoritative. They do, however, have a number of disadvantages. The information they contain has been filtered, it is affected by the perhaps well-concealed prejudices of the author, and many authors make assertions without making it clear on what evidence these are based. Wyatt writes that in the *Oxford Handbook of Medicine* only 1% of the details are referenced[14].

The chief problem with textbooks, however, is that they are often out of date. Indeed this is inevitable, given that they can take many months if not years to write and at least an additional 6 months to bring to market. This is not to take into account the delay between the original publication of clinical evidence and its inclusion in standard textbooks. Antman *et al.* discovered that the routine use of streptokinase in myocardial infarction began to be advised in textbooks only in 1987, 13 years after a meta-analysis of clinical trials would have revealed clear and compelling evidence to support it[15].

The limitations of book publishing are partly to do with the generation of content. They are also, in part, to do with the mechanics of both production and dissemination. The cost of printing, binding, distributing, selling and storing volumes of bound pages means that books are updated infrequently and tend to stay on the purchaser's shelves for years if not decades.

Electronic access to books

There are various ways in which new technology can enable content published in book form to be updated more easily. The earliest attempts at electronic publication involved distributing books on CDROM and this format still has advantages. The software used in conjunction with the CDROM allows the reader to navigate through the material in different ways, especially if comprehensive indices have been compiled. This can seem a great advantage in theory but has to be weighed up against the advantages of traditional forms of publication. We are used to navigating our way through books and have highly evolved strategies for reading, skimming, searching and browsing and can take advantage of a range of cues about information implicit in the design and presentation of books. The real advantage of CDROMs is that the marginal cost of 'printing' a CDROM is extremely low compared to that of a traditional book, particularly a large textbook, and so it becomes easier to supply a purchaser with frequent updates.

It is even more straightforward to issue subscribers with the latest version of a book if the medium of publication is the Web. But although the Web has transformed the way many of us access medical journals, very few medical textbooks have been published via the Web. The economics of the Web have tended to mitigate this (although this may change with the advent of 'wiki-books', as explained below). 'ebooks' are now being sold through the Web, however. An ebook is simply a formatted textfile, generally downloaded, on payment of a purchase fee, from the Internet to a portable digital assistant (PDA), such as a Palm Pilot.

Accessing www.ebooks.com on 17 March 2005, I found 1707 books listed under the heading 'medical'. Not all of these, by any means, were aimed at clinicians but many specialist and sub-specialist reference works were included. An example relevant to the case of Isabel Maude is: Ahrens W, Strange G *et al. Pediatric Emergency Medicine: Companion Handbook*, McGraw-Hill. This volume 'covers the essentials of clinical signs, pathophysiology, diagnosis and treatment of all pediatric emergencies commonly seen in the emergency department (ED) or the primary care setting. The outline format makes access to critical information quick and easy.' The advantage of ebooks is chiefly that they are exceptionally portable. A single PDA can store many textbooks and still work as a personal organiser. The disadvantages are that only a limited number of books are currently available in this form, and many of those are in editions aimed at the US market. The limited screen size and resolution of PDAs also constrains the way the texts can be displayed and read.

One of the recent developments on the Web is the 'wiki'. Wikipedia defines a wiki as 'a website (or other hypertext document collection) that allows users to add content, as on an Internet forum, but also allows anyone to edit the content'[16]. The central idea is that all the content is available to be edited by anyone with access to the Web. This requires, first, that easy-to-use editing software be available to allow naive users to contribute. Second, there must be a clear system with a set of templates to ensure that the diverse contributions form an integrated whole with a reasonably consistent house style. Third, there must be an effective mechanism for correcting errors.

The term wiki, which comes from the 'wiki wiki' or 'quick' shuttle buses at Honolulu Airport, was picked by Ward Cunningham, who came up with the idea in the early 1990s. Wiki technology was used as the basis for an electronic encyclopedia, Wikipedia, launched in January 2001. Today, it is the world's largest wiki containing almost half a million articles (as of 17 March 2005). Other public wikis are listed at WorldWideWiki. The wiki concept is also being used to allow authors to collaborate on open-access textbooks. This movement is in its infancy but already medical textbooks are being put together.

Journals

Publication in scientific and medical journals is the usual way to disseminate new ideas, experimental results or analytical findings. Journal articles are up to date (although it is worth noting that the process of peer-reviewed publication can take a year or so, and the data discussed may have taken several years to collect), comprehensive and widely available. They are not, however, ideal as an information source for the busy clinician. First, there are more than 5000 medical journals published worldwide every month. There are more than 15 million medical articles on library shelves[17]. Even with the tools now available for searching databases of published articles, the sheer scale of the medical literature is inevitably discouraging.

A vast majority of published articles are read by only a handful of readers in the same field, cited once or twice at best before they disappear into the archives. It is neither cynical nor controversial to say that the primary motive for publication is career progression and so a great many unnecessary articles are published.

The presence of a great deal of dross is not the only difficulty facing a clinician who tries to answer a question by using the primary research literature. Many, if not most, of the articles are written as contributions to clinical research rather than as attempts to help clinical decision-making. This means that even when the information in the article is genuinely useful, it is often written up and presented in such a way that a practising clinician will struggle to find it.

Electronic access to journals

Most medical journals are now available in an electronic form. PubMed provides an easy interface to a comprehensive list of published articles, many of which are accessible, in their electronic form, via a link from the PubMed search engine. Researchers and practising clinicians can therefore get at the literature from anywhere with Internet access, subject to a financial constraint: the electronic forms of journals are available only to people who can either identify themselves as subscribers or who are prepared to pay a fee for one-off access. Free access is generally restricted to employees of organisations who have paid some form of subscription, perhaps the cost of an institutional subscription to the paper form of the journal.

The economics of academic publishing are a little different from those of conventional publishing in that the content is not paid for by the publisher. Neither the author nor the funding body that paid for the research therefore have any interest in restricting the readership to those who are prepared to pay for it. Research organisations are now considering alternatives to traditional journal publication, which might provide cheaper access to research findings. The problem is that journals perform a number of functions in addition to the obvious one of the dissemination of research; they provide a form of quality control. One alternative to traditional journal publication is to set up an organisation that can play the same role as a traditional journal – sub-editing, ensuring peer review and publicising journal content – but which is supported financially by the organisations that fund research, with the consequence that the content can be made freely available and copyright retained by the author. Biomed Central is one such organisation, hosting a number of open-access journals[18].

New forms of clinical information

Systematic reviews

It is tempting, given how difficult it is to find practical advice in journal publications, for the busy reader simply to ignore the primary literature. This has led to a growing demand for what is termed 'secondary literature'. A number of specialist journals, databases and websites now publish critical reviews of the evidence relating to common questions. If, for example, I want to know whether angiotensin converting enzyme inhibitors improve outcomes following acute myocardial infarction, I could go to PubMed, type in *angiotensin converting enzyme inhibitors* and *acute myocardial infarction*. This search identifies 1982 articles, 370 of which are clinical trials published in English. Sifting through this evidence to come to an informed decision would take a long time. One alternative would be to consult a site organised like the *BMJ's Clinical Evidence* at http://www.clinicalevidence.com. Navigating through a hierarchical structure leading from cardiovascular disorders to acute myocardial infarction to *benefits from angiotensin converting enzyme inhibitors* leads to a summary of the available evidence.

> One overview and one systematic review in people within 36 hours of acute myocardial infarction have found that angiotensin converting enzyme inhibitors versus placebo significantly reduce mortality. The overview also found that angiotensin converting enzyme inhibitors versus control significantly increase persistent hypotension and renal dysfunction. The question of whether angiotensin converting enzyme inhibitors should be offered to everyone presenting with acute myocardial infarction or only to people with signs of heart failure remains unresolved.[19]

The reader is referred to the two reviews, one published in *Circulation* and the other in the *Journal of the American College of Cardiologists*. More information is also given on the evidence about the benefits and dangers of this treatment and there are remarks about the form further research should take.

A systematic review, like the one referred to in the quotation, is an attempt by a small team or even an individual to assemble all the published, or even unpublished, evidence relating to a well-defined question. To do this it is necessary to trawl the databases of published research – such as PubMed – and identify trials or research funding that may have led to unpublished research. Such trials are then appraised, first to confirm that they are relevant to the question under review, and next to find out whether they meet agreed standards of scientific rigour. The studies that meet the criteria are analysed, classified and categorised so that the results can be published as an overview, which makes it easy to see whether the available evidence provides an answer to the original question. The systematic review is one of the key elements in the practice of evidence-based medicine, as described in Chapter 1.

One of the prime movers in encouraging people to carry out systematic reviews of the evidence relating to a particular question has been the Cochrane Collaboration, an international non-profit and independent organisation founded in 1993 and named after the epidemiologist, Archie Cochrane[20]. Its site at http://www.cochrane.org contains not just abstracts of the systematic reviews relating to literally hundreds of common clinical questions but also guides describing how to carry out systematic reviews and appraise clinical evidence.

Clinical guidelines

Initiatives such as the Cochrane Collaboration want to allow new research findings to change clinical practice more quickly. Other sites try to alter clinical practice by publishing clinical guidelines or protocols for the treatment of particular conditions. At first glance this approach might seem unduly prescriptive, and it has been criticised on these grounds. But guidelines do not have to be prescriptive, and a clinical guideline could be pretty much the same as a user-friendly presentation of the results of a systematic review. One good, reputable source of evidence-based guidelines is the Scottish Intercollegiate Guideline Network, which can be found at http://www.sign. ac.uk/.

As well as publishing clinical guidelines, in both a summarised and comprehensive form, the website explains the methodology used to develop the guidelines[21]. The methodology for SIGN guidelines is based on three key principles:
- Development is carried out by multidisciplinary, nationally representative groups.
- A systematic review is conducted to identify and critically appraise the evidence.
- Recommendations are explicitly linked to the supporting evidence.

Box 4.1 shows the criteria used to grade the evidence on which the different categories of recommendation are based.

The term 'guideline' can, however, be used to refer to a variety of things, and that is one of the problems with clinical guidelines: there are an enormous number of them, produced and disseminated by different bodies and not all of them are grounded in clinical evidence, and even when they are, this is not always well documented. Hibble *et al.* published a short but engaging article describing guidelines as the 'new Tower of Babel'[22]. In a survey of 22 general practices they found 855 clinical guidelines, a stack of paper weighing 28 kg. Clearly the impact of any one guideline is going to be limited because it is competing for the GPs' attention with a multiplicity of others. The authors write that we should consider electronic means for disseminating guidelines.

A systematic review of evaluations of attempts to change practice seems to show that guidelines are effective[23]. The assessment of the comparative effectiveness of different attempts to change clinical practice has shown that

Box 4.1 A set of criteria used to grade levels of clinical evidence and appropriate recommendations

Statements of evidence:

Ia   Evidence obtained from meta-analysis of randomised controlled trials.

Ib   Evidence obtained from at least one randomised controlled trial.

IIa   Evidence obtained from at least one well-designed controlled study without randomisation.

IIb   Evidence obtained from at least one other type of well-designed quasi-experimental study.

III   Evidence obtained from well-designed non-experimental descriptive studies, such as comparative studies, correlation studies and case studies.

IV   Evidence obtained from expert committee reports or opinions and/or clinical experiences of respected authorities.

Grades of recommendations:

A   Requires at least one randomised controlled trial as part of a body of literature of overall good quality and consistency addressing the specific recommendation (evidence levels Ia, Ib).

B   Requires the availability of well-conducted clinical studies but no randomised clinical trials on the topic of recommendation (evidence levels IIa, IIb, III).

C   Requires evidence obtained from expert committee reports or opinions and/or clinical experiences of respected authorities. Indicates an absence of directly applicable clinical studies of good quality (evidence level IV).

no method is always successful and that passive information interventions (such as mailing a guideline to GPs) are unlikely to work. The question then arises of whether guidelines can be used actively, to generate reminders of the appropriate course of action. This can be achieved if guidelines are disseminated electronically as part of a decision support system.

Decision support systems

The first decision support systems were created as a result of research into what were called expert systems. The idea was that you could build computer systems that would represent the facts used in making diagnoses and implement the algorithms used in clinical reasoning. It was assumed that the superior storage and processing capacities of a computer would allow it to perform as well as an expert.

One of the best-known decision support systems was the Quick Medical Reference system, which was based on an earlier research project: Internist-1[24].

The research project was taken up and turned into a commercial product by one of the more successful companies dealing in health knowledge and information. The system contained a knowledge base of facts of about 600 diseases and 4500 clinical findings used in their diagnosis[25]. Users of the system would start by entering an initial set of clinical findings describing their patient's case. These findings were then used by the system to generate hypotheses. The user could then review the hypothesis set and enter further findings and test results in pursuit of different diagnostic strategies, for example, to try and rule out alternative diagnosis or to increase the evidence in favour of the preferred hypothesis.

The hypotheses would be diseases that, according to the knowledge base, were associated with the entered findings. The system calculated a score for each hypothesis. The calculation was a complex one; it took into account not just the strength of the association between each of the entered findings and the disease but also the number of findings that would be explained by the hypothesis, the number of findings that it failed to explain and the number of other findings that would have been expected, but which were absent.

The knowledge base of quality media resources (QMR) consisted of two sets of facts linking findings and diseases. One recorded the evoking strength, which was a subjective measure of likelihood of the disease given the symptom. A sign with an evoking strength of 0 would be completely non-specific while a sign with an evoking strength of 5 would always suggest the disease. The other set of facts, termed frequency, was a subjective measure of the likelihood of the symptom given the disease. A sign rarely seen with a disease was given a frequency of 1 and a sign seen in essentially all cases was given a frequency of 5 for the disease. For example, red hair is found in about half of the patients with skin cancer, and would therefore have a score of 3 for frequency. Nevertheless, if a patient has red hair, that in itself is not sufficient to suggest that he or she has skin cancer, so the sign would have an evoking strength of 0 for skin cancer: completely non-specific. QMR used the ratings of frequency and evoking strength for the findings entered by the user to derive a score for each possible explanation of an entered finding; a threshold on the scores would determine which of the competing explanations made it into the hypothesis set.

The success of the system was therefore critically dependent on the accuracy and completeness of the ratings making up the knowledge base, which in turn meant that the system's developers had to give a great deal of thought to the process by which the ratings were obtained and kept up to date. The procedure followed in developing, extending and updating the system was organised around the notion of a disease profile, a list of 25–250 findings associated with the disease. The knowledge base was extended through the addition of new disease profiles. The creation of a profile involved, first, a search of the relevant textbooks and research literature and next consultation with relevant experts. The results were then reviewed by the QMR project team and tested with 'classic' cases.

A number of evaluations of QMR have been published. There are no RCTs in which the outcomes for patients treated by doctors using the system are compared to those of patients treated by doctors not using the system. It is probably not realistic to expect a tool of this kind to have an impact that could be measured in that way. Broadly speaking, assessments of QMR have fallen into one of two categories: some have looked at the accuracy of the suggestions generated by the tool; others have looked at the impact of those suggestions on clinicians' decision-making. Although some studies use cases derived from real life, all were carried out as 'laboratory' experiments in which users had to use the system rather than field trials, in which they were free to choose when to use it. Almost all involved users working with sets of notes or scenarios described by the experimenter, rather than actual living and breathing patients.

Assessments of the system's accuracy generally measured the percentage of cases in which the 'correct' diagnosis is one of the first five hypotheses generated by the system. What counts as 'correct' is of course a tricky issue. Graber and VanScoy looked at 25 patients who presented to the ED with a diagnostic question and found that when the patient data collected in the ED was entered into QMR, the correct hypothesis was in the top five 32% of the time[26]. They defined correct as being the final diagnosis when the patient left the ED, which they concede may not have been the true diagnosis. Lemaire *et al.* reviewed the notes for 1144 cases treated in a tertiary hospital and identified 154 patients referred for an undiagnosed disease and for whom a final definitive diagnosis was obtained[27]. They took from the notes the information available at the time of referral and entered it into QMR. The correct response was generated, as a top five hypothesis, 38% of the time. The authors found that it was able to identify rare diseases correctly, for example, suggesting thoracic actinomycosis as the diagnosis for a patient with the following findings: fluctuant chest-wall mass, cough, fever, chest pain, dyspnoea and hoarseness, leukocytosis and anaemia, and a chest radiograph showing a pleural mass, nodules and hilar densities. The system fared less well on non-specific presentations. One of the patients in the study was a 42-year-old woman with a 10-day history of nausea, myalgia, fever and chills, headache, pain in the lower abdominal region and anorexia and also hepatomegaly, leukocytosis, mild anaemia and a tender abdomen. In this case the correct diagnosis, tubo-ovarian abscess, was the 156th suggestion.

At least one published trial of the system found that it was an effective tool in influencing clinical decision-making, although perhaps of greater benefit to students and junior doctors than their more experienced colleagues. Friedman *et al.* recruited 216 clinicians who each reviewed 9 of 36 paper cases, and recorded a differential diagnosis set before and after using either QMR or a competitor[28]. They were rated on the crude measure of whether or not the 'correct' diagnosis was included in the set but also on a specially designed measure of diagnostic quality. The quality score combined a measure of the plausibility of each component listed with a score for the ranking given to the correct score. The correct diagnosis was generated by the software in 40% of cases. The correct diagnosis figured in users' differential diagnosis sets on 39% of occasions before using QMR and on 46% of occasions after QMR. The mean score for diagnostic quality went up from 5.6 to 6.2 when the system was used.

However, QMR has now been suspended from sales. The last software version ran on Windows 98 systems. The knowledge base is still owned by First Databank and was last updated at the end of 2002. In the long run, the system has met the same fate as AAPHelp. The market for decision support tools is an uncertain one. It is not clear exactly what we should conclude from past failures. A newer version of QMR marketed via the Web and available for use on a PDA might well prove a more successful product. Tools that provide the same kind of assistance are being developed, although they are generally developed more as aids for accessing information about diseases rather than as tools to help in decision-making.

Guideline-based decision support

Hunt *et al.* published a systematic review of clinical trials of decision support systems, which found clear evidence for the effectiveness of such systems, with 43 out of 65 trials showing an improvement in physician performance[29]. Perhaps the most telling finding in their review, however, was that only five of those trials had been carried out for diagnostic decision aids and, of them, only one had shown an effect. It was an unstated assumption of the pioneers of expert systems that diagnosis was the decision on which such systems should concentrate. The assumption seemed to have been false, although a more recent review found ten trials of diagnostic systems of which four had a positive result[30]. Nineteen of the systems reviewed by Hunt *et al.* were described as preventive care or reminder systems and 14 of them were found to have been effective. For example, Safran *et al.* described a controlled trial of a computer-based patient record system that generated messages to alert clinicians to events specified in guidelines for human immunodeficiency virus (HIV) care. They found greatly improved response times[31]. Pestotnik *et al.* carried out a careful study of the use of decision support systems with guidelines, put together by local clinicians, for antibiotic therapy[32]. They found that the use of antibiotics was better targeted, costs were reduced and the emergence of antibiotic-resistant pathogens stabilised.

The Isabel decision aid

The Isabel Medical Charity wanted to build a system of the sort that the early developers of expert systems had envisaged, one that would help with diagnosis. The decision aid at the centre of the Isabel site works, at least in broad terms, in the same way as QMR: you enter a set of symptoms and it suggests possible diagnoses. The two systems, however, work in entirely different ways. Essentially Isabel works like an Internet search engine[33]. In QMR, the computer contains a set of facts about the way symptoms relate to diseases and an algorithm that, given a set of symptoms, can use these facts to identify a set of plausible diseases. In Isabel, the system contains a set of texts describing diseases and an algorithm that, given a set of symptoms, can identify the set of texts that describe the most likely diseases.

I said earlier on that searching a database of research such as PubMed – which like Isabel is made up of a set of texts – using a set of symptoms as keywords would not return a set of articles describing possible diagnoses. But there are two key differences between PubMed and Isabel. The first is the nature of the textual content: Isabel contains text fragments that were obtained by dividing standard paediatric textbooks into sections, one disease per section. The second is that Isabel does not have a standard search engine but uses software supplied by a company called Autonomy. According to the company's website: 'Autonomy's software identifies the patterns that naturally occur in text, based on the usage and frequency of words or terms that correspond to specific ideas or concepts. Based on the preponderance of one pattern over another in a piece of unstructured information, Autonomy enables computers to understand that there is $x\%$ of probability that a document in question is about a specific subject'[34]. We come back to Bayes' theorem.

The system is still being evaluated and it remains to be seen whether the approach will fare any better than QMR. Even if it does not, it is likely to be influential. More and more effort is going into the development of search tools capable of identifying documents by analysing their content and creating a model of the user's preferences. Autonomy's software works on the basis of an analysis of textual patterns, probably looking at the frequency with which different combinations of words occur in fragments at different distances apart. Other researchers are looking at tools that have a more explicit model of language and the roles different words play. For example, PASTA is a database of papers on molecular biology that can be accessed via a query system that combines domain knowledge with the automated interpretation of texts[35]. It is likely that text-retrieval systems will come to be used in much the same way as decision support systems. These systems will use techniques of analysis and reasoning that have been developed through research into the artificial intelligence, where the original work on expert systems started.

Conclusions

No single clinician's experience can provide an adequate basis for making decisions about treatment or diagnosis. The mechanisms we use to share knowledge drawn from the experience of others now generate such an excess of information that we need to reflect on how best to use it to answer clinical questions.

Attempts to use computers to solve the information problem in health care began with the development of expert systems and continued with the development of decision support systems. These proved least effective where they were first thought to be most needed, in helping with diagnosis. They have, however, proved effective as tools for the dissemination of clinical guidelines; indeed it is argued that such guidelines are most likely to be effective if they are computerised.

Attempts to address the information problem have led to the development of evidence-based medicine and of databases containing systematic reviews. The Internet and the World Wide Web mean that these databases are now readily accessible to clinicians. This ease of access is bound to increase as computers become smaller and more widely used. Creating more intelligent tools for accessing these databases will also help clinical decision-making.

There are those who argue that findings from published research are implemented so slowly in clinical practice not because there is an 'information deficit' problem but rather a 'behaviour change' problem. On this interpretation the difficulty is not about getting the information to practitioners but creating the conditions that enable them to change their practice. Poses *et al.* found that improving clinicians' understanding of the deficiencies in their own decision-making failed to change their behaviour[36]. Macfarlane *et al.* attempted an educational programme aimed at reducing inappropriate prescription of antibiotics by GPs[37]. When this did not work, they looked more carefully at the problem and discovered that GPs' prescribing behaviour, in this area at least, was not determined by what they thought was correct but by what they thought their patients expected. The authors then designed a patient information leaflet, which helped reduce the demand for inappropriate prescriptions. Later chapters look at not just how to build tools that can get information to clinicians but how to take into account the setting in which they are to be used.

References

1. Meikle J. Parents invest in aid to NHS. *The Guardian*, 18 June 2002.
2. Pollard AJ, Isaacs A, Lyall HEG, *et al.* Potentially lethal bacterial infection associated with varicella zoster virus. *BMJ* 1996;313(7052):283–285.
3. Ely JW, Burch RJ, Vinson DC. The information needs of family physicians: case-specific clinical questions. *J Fam Pract* 1992;35(3):265–269.
4. Covell DG, Uman GC, Manning PR. Information needs in office practice: are they being met? *Ann Intern Med* 1985;103(4):596–599.
5. Weinberg AD, Ullian L, Richards WD, Cooper C. Informal advice and information seeking between physicians. *J Med Educ* 1981;56:174–180.
6. Coiera E, Tombs V. Communication behaviours in a hospital setting: an observational study. *BMJ* 1998;316:673–676.
7. Wenger E, McDermott R, Snyder WM. *Cultivating Communities of Practice*. Boston: Harvard Business School Press, 2002.
8. Crippen D. Critical care and the Internet: a clinician's perspective. *Crit Care Clin* 1999;5:604–614.
9. Ward MF. Developing a mental health network to support research. *Nurse Res* 2000;7:3–24.

10. Wootton R, Craig J. *Introduction to Telemedicine*. London: RSM Press, 1999.
11. May C, Harrison R, MacFarlane A, Williams T, Mair F, Wallace P. Why do telemedicine systems fail to normalize as stable models of service delivery? *J Telemed Telecare* 2003;9 (Suppl 1):S25–S26.
12. May C, Gask L, Atkinson T, Ellis N, Mair F, Esmail A. Resisting and promoting new technologies in clinical practice: the case of telepsychiatry. *Soc Sci Med* 2001; 52(12):1889–1901.
13. Roine R, Ohinmaa A, Hailey D. Assessing telemedicine: a systematic review of the literature. *CMAJ* 2001;165(6):765–771.
14. Wyatt J. Use and sources of medical knowledge. *Lancet* 1991;338:1368–1373.
15. Antman EM, Lau J, Kupelnick B, Mosteller F, Chalmers TC. Comparison of results of meta-analyses of randomized control trials and recommendations of clinical experts: treatments for myocardial infarction. *JAMA* 1992;268(2):240A–248A.
16. Wikipedia *Wiki*. http://en.wikipedia.org/wiki/Wiki (accessed on 17 March 2005).
17. Smith R. What clinical information do doctors need? *BMJ* 1996;313:1062–1068.
18. BioMed Central. *What is BioMed Central?* http://www.biomedcentral.com/info/ (accessed on 17 March 2005).
19. McKelvie R. Heart failure: angiotensin converting enzyme inhibitors. *Clinical Evidence* 2004. http://www.clinicalevidence.com/ceweb/conditions/cvd/0204/0204_I3. jsp (accessed on 17 March 2005).
20. The Cochrane Collaboration. *What is the Cochrane Collaboration?* http://www. cochrane.org/ docs/descrip.htm (accessed on 17 March 2005).
21. Scottish Intercollegiate Guideline Network Sign 50: A guideline developer's handbook http://www.sign.ac.uk/guidelines/fulltext/50/ index.html (accessed on 17 March 2005).
22. Hibble A, Kanka D, Pencheon D, Pooles F. Guidelines in general practice: the new Tower of Babel? *BMJ* 1998;317(7162):862–863.
23. Grimshaw JM, Thomas RE, MacLennan G, Fraser C, Ramsay CR, Vale L, Whitty P, Eccles MP, Matowe L, Shirran L, Wensing M, Dijkstra R, Donaldson C. Effectiveness and efficiency of guideline dissemination and implementation strategies. *Health Technol Assess* 2004;8(6):iii–iv, 1–72.
24. Miller RA, Pople HE, Myers J. Internist 1. an experimental computer-based diagnostic consultant for general internal medicine. *N Engl J Med* 1982;307:468–476.
25. Giuse DA, Giuse NB, Miller RA. Evaluation of long-term maintenance of a large medical knowledge base. *J Am Med Inform Assoc* 1995;2(5):297–306.
26. Graber MA, VanScoy D. How well does decision support software perform in the emergency department? *Emerg Med J* 2003;20(5):426–428.
27. Lemaire JB, Schaefer JP, Martin LA, Faris P, Ainslie MD, Hull RD. Effectiveness of the Quick Medical Reference as a diagnostic tool. *CMAJ* 1999;161(6):725–728.
28. Friedman CP, Elstein AS, Wolf FM, *et al*. Enhancements of clinicians' diagnostic reasoning by computer-based consultation. *JAMA* 1999;282:1851–1856.
29. Hunt DL, Haynes RB, Hanna SE, Smith K. Effects of computer-based clinical decision support systems on physician performance and patient outcomes: a systematic review. *JAMA* 1998;280:1339–1346.
30. Garg AX, Adhikari NK, McDonald H, *et al*. Effects of computerized clinical decision support systems on practitioner performance and patient outcomes: a systematic review. *JAMA* 2005; 293(10):1223–1238.
31. Safran C, Rind DM, Davis RB, *et al*. Guidelines for management of HIV infection with computer-based patient records. *Lancet* 1995;346:341–346.

32. Pestotnik SL, Classen DC, Evans RS, Burke JP. Implementing antibiotic practice guidelines through computer-assisted decision support: clinical and financial outcomes. *Ann Intern Med* 1996;124:884–890.

33. Ramnarayan P, Britto J. Paediatric clinical decision support systems. *Arch Dis Child* 2002;87(5):361–362.

34. Autonomy Technology Introduction. http://www.autonomy.com/content/Technology/ (accessed on 17 March 2005).

35. Gaizauskas R, Demetriou G, Artymiuk PJ, Willett P. Protein structures and information extraction from biological texts: the PASTA system. *Bioinformatics* 2003;19:135–143.

36. Poses RM, Cebul RD, Wigton RS. You can lead a horse to water – improving physicians' knowledge of probabilities may not affect their decisions. *Med Decis Making* 1995;15:65–75.

37. Macfarlane J, Holmes W, Gard P, *et al*. Reducing antibiotic use for acute bronchitis in primary care: blinded, randomised controlled trial of patient information leaflet. *BMJ* 2002;324:91.

Part 2
The Principles of Health Informatics

CHAPTER 5
Representation

The goals of health informatics

Part 1 described three grand challenges for health informatics: improving the recording and organisation of patient data, using data in research and, finally, ensuring that the knowledge so gained is used to best effect. A variety of tools will be required to meet these challenges: electronic health care records that allow the sharing of information between different institutions; systems that can find patients who fit the inclusion criteria for new clinical trials and decision support tools capable of checking prescriptions in order to avoid allergies and dangerous combinations of drugs.

There are technical and practical problems here, but there is also a compelling intellectual problem, one which has bedevilled research in this field for decades, and which is of such subtlety that it is often quite hard to see that there is a problem at all. It is certainly not obvious precisely how to characterise it; it could be described as the problem of representing 'meanings'. It is, essentially, the subject of this chapter.

Imagine that a patient goes to see his or her GP with a set of symptoms suggestive of diabetes. The GP records the patient's history and adds '?Diab'. Later, when the test results come back, the record is amended to say 'Dx confirmed'. The doctor's meaning is absolutely clear: the patient has been recorded as having diabetes. In fact the meaning is so clear that it is a shock to realise just how hard it would be to write a program that was able to analyse the record and identify this patient as a diabetic. The program would have to do more than just recognise the abbreviations; it would have to identify the role of the first statement as a particular kind of observation about the patient (a provisional diagnosis) and the second statement not as a new statement about the patient, but a modification of the earlier one. We are so good at seeing the meanings behind written or spoken words that it is actually quite difficult to work out precisely what we have to do to get from the words to the meanings.

Programming computers to understand language

If you watch an old sci-fi movie, like Stanley Kubrick's *2001: A Space Odyssey*, you can see how misguided people's expectations of the development of computers were. Computers in the 1960s were rare, large and expensive items and had fairly limited capabilities. At the time, people imagined that computers now would still be rare, large and expensive but would rival human beings not just in their capacity to perform calculations but also in their capacity for intelligent thought, interpretation of language and sensory perception. As we know, computers now are incredibly small, relatively cheap and therefore astonishingly common. But they are pretty poor at performing many tasks humans are good at, the use of language being a prime example. In terms of intelligence, our computers are closer to those of the 1960s than they are to HAL.

Why was it so much harder than people expected to develop intelligent software? Consider one specific aspect of intelligent behaviour: that involved in understanding language. Part of what we do when we interpret language is to identify the concepts or ideas that words represent. Researchers sometimes talk about understanding language as though it is a process of translation, from the language of words into the language of thought. Broadly speaking, there are two views as to the reason it seems difficult to program computers to do this: first, it seems difficult because it is difficult; and second, it seems difficult because, actually, it is impossible.

The 'Cyc' project

A well-known researcher in the difficult-but-doable camp is Doug Lenat, who takes the view that we can interpret language only by bringing to bear an enormous amount of knowledge, particularly the sort we acquire effortlessly as a consequence of being the kind of creature that grows up surrounded by, and communicating with, others. This knowledge is not so much of the sort you find in the encyclopaedia as of the knowledge you need to have to be able to read the encyclopaedia. The point is that an encyclopaedia's authors will assume that you already know that trees are usually outdoors, that once people die they stop buying things and that glasses of liquid should be carried the right way up. It is almost impossible to imagine the range and scope of such knowledge, but that does not mean, at least not in Lenat's eyes, that it cannot, eventually, be elucidated, rendered explicit and represented on a computer. And that is exactly what he is attempting to do, in a project called 'Cyc'. Critics of the project argue that it is not enough simply to possess this kind of knowledge; one has to know which bits are relevant, and this involves a different, intuitive knowledge, something more akin to possessing a skill than to being aware of a fact. It is worth noting that although the initial R&D project is now over and the Cyc Corporation has a website that advertises commercial products, it does not seem to have transformed the way in which we interact with computers[1].

The Chinese Room argument

The argument that computers will never understand language has been put forward by a number of philosophers over the years, one of the best known being John Searle. On his account, understanding is not a matter of manipulating symbols but rather of being sensitive to the meaning of those symbols.

He would argue that even if one could automate a process of translation from one set of symbols to another, it would not help because some other kind of process is needed to move from symbols to understanding.

He uses a powerful thought experiment to get his ideas across[2]. Imagine that someone is in a room with a large book and a stack of tablets on which Chinese characters have been inscribed. The room has two windows. More tablets of Chinese characters are being passed in through the first window and, for each sequence of characters passed in, the book lists a sequence of characters to be passed out through the second window. The person in the room has to collect the tablets as they are passed in, look the characters up in the book and then pass the appropriate tablets out. Imagine that the book is so well designed and so comprehensive that the illusion is maintained that the person in the room understands Chinese. Searle's point is that this would be an illusion. Most people would not want to say that the person or the book or the room or the person-book-and-room together understands Chinese. It would seem to follow, from this, that understanding must involve something other than manipulating symbols according to predefined rules, which is, classically, all that a computer can do.

Representing meanings

It is clear, therefore, that after 40 years of research, we are still a long way from computers capable of making effective use of ordinary language and that there are powerful, if contentious, arguments to the effect that understanding is an intrinsically human capacity. Given all this, one should perhaps be sceptical about the potential for computers to interpret language. Health informatics, of course, does not require the creation of computers capable of understanding natural language, but it does require computer systems that can represent concepts rooted in human experience, and many of the same issues apply.

One of the major aims of health informatics is the development of clinical decision support tools integrated with the patient record. The idea is to codify the knowledge used to make decisions on diagnoses, treatment and so forth, and represent it in terms of rules that can be automatically tested against the contents of computer-based records. This would be easy if the rules could be tested against patient histories simply by checking if the words used in these rules are present in the histories. The problem occurs when the rule to be tested contains a condition, say 'a tumour of more than 1 cm in diameter' and the record contains a statement that matches the condition but that is expressed in a completely different way, e.g. 'palpable lump in left breast'. We want to find a way of representing the meaning underlying the words, so that the statement in the rule matches that in the record. But representing 'meaning' in a computer is exactly what we do not seem able to do.

Much of the research in health informatics aims to build systems that circumvent this problem. There are two ways of doing this: one is to build systems that do not need to represent 'meanings' in this way; the other is to capitalise on the extent to which scientific medicine is a formalised body of knowledge and, therefore, one that *can* be analysed, codified and represented in computer programs. A great deal of the work in health informatics involves trying to exploit the inherent structure in medical knowledge in order to build representations that can capture enough of the meaning of clinical terms to allow us to build computer systems that work well enough to be useful. The rest of this chapter looks more closely at the idea of representation, and the way information is represented in computer software. First, we will analyse the most straightforward form of representation: pictures.

Pictorial representations

Consider an X-ray image and the process by which it is created. To take an X-ray, a body is positioned between an X-ray source and a sheet of X-ray film. The film records the pattern created by the X-rays that pass through the body. This pattern contains information about the body because the tissues in the body absorb some of the X-rays, and some kinds of tissue absorb more than others. Bone absorbs more X-rays than soft tissue and so a region of X-ray film that lies behind a bone will be exposed to fewer photons than one lying behind soft tissue. Such a region will show up as white when the film is developed. The arrangement of light and dark on the film provides information about the arrangement of different tissues in the body. We can say that the image represents or depicts the tissues, or, more correctly, it depicts the radio-absorbent properties of the imaged tissues (Figures 5.1 and 5.2). The image conveys information about the anatomy because the process by which the image was created ensures that anatomical properties are directly observable in the image (see Box 5.1).

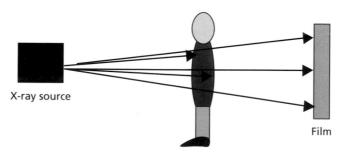

Figure 5.1 An X-ray image of a body is created by positioning the body between a camera and a film. Some of the photons are absorbed by the body, others pass through, creating a pattern of light and dark regions on the film that corresponds to the X-ray absorbent properties of the body.

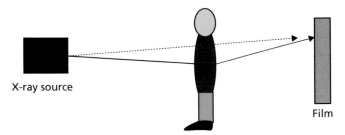

Figure 5.2 Some photons are deflected as they pass through the body. These 'scattered photons' create errors or 'noise' in the image since they are interpreted as having passed through the body in a straight line.

Box 5.1 Molecular imaging

We see the world as we do because the photoreceptive cells in our retinas respond to light reflected from the surfaces of the objects around us and, in doing so, tell us something about how those surfaces are arranged in space. The extraordinary thing about X-ray imaging is that X-ray film responds to radiation that has passed through certain materials, so X-rays tell us about things we cannot see, things that lie behind the visible surfaces. We can use X-rays to create a variety of different kinds of image. Computed tomography (CT) uses X-rays to create a set of images of slices through a patient, a stack of which can then be assembled by computer into a 3D image. Each slice is created by rotating an X-ray source around the patient's body, capturing a large number of measurements of transmitted X-rays for points on the circumference. Each measurement is then used as an estimate of the pixel values for all the points along the ray between the X-ray source and detector, i.e. along a line through the centre of the circle. Back-projecting in this way for each measurement allows an image to be built up. It is as though the X-ray measurement is a quantity of ink that is then smeared back, drawing an even line, and as more and more lines are added, a picture gradually emerges.

There are disadvantages to using X-rays in medical imaging, not least of which is that X-ray photons have sufficient energy to dislodge electrons from molecules in the body, a large enough dose of X-rays can so interfere with the body's chemistry that cancerous tumours may develop. Images can also be created using ultrasound, very high-frequency sound waves that are partially reflected at the boundaries between acoustically distinct materials (unlike with X-rays, ultrasound images are created from the reflected, not the transmitted, signal). Another approach, which can be used to build 3D images, is to detect the

(continued)

Box 5.1 Molecular imaging (*continued*)

radio-frequency pulse emitted when the magnetic dipoles of protons of hydrogen atoms are placed in a magnetic field alternating at the resonant frequency of the dipoles. Magnetic resonance imaging (MRI) can be used to build up true 3D images of anatomy. By setting up gradients in the strength of the magnetic field along the z-axis, in the frequency of the pulse along the y-axis and the phase of the pulse along the x-axis, we can ensure that a signal can be assigned to a precise location in the 3D space. The emitted signal is determined by a combination of factors concerning, for example, the rate at which excited protons give up energy to the surrounding molecular lattice. By adjusting the way in which the signal is obtained, different images can be obtained that are weighted to bring out the contrast between different tissue types.

MRI is a highly sophisticated technique providing 3D images of the body. One particularly exciting application involves capturing a sequence of MRI images of the brain, say 30 complete images acquired over a period of 90 s. The changes between the images tell us something about what the brain is doing. Neural activity in a region of the brain increases blood flow in that region and increased blood flow lowers the concentration of deoxyhaemoglobin, and deoxyhaemoglobin is paramagnetic, which means it alters the contrast of the MRI image. The result is what we call a functional image: an image which is of interest not for the information it contains about the shape and arrangement of our internal organs, but for the information it gives us about how they are behaving. Our ability to create such images has revolutionised experimental neuroscience: it is now possible to perform studies in which we record the effect on neural activity of performing different cognitive tasks.

Functional MRI (fMRI) is not the only modality that allows us to create functional images. Another technique, which is also used extensively in neuroscience is positron emission tomography (PET). This is a form of nuclear medicine study, which means that the image is created by detecting particles emitted from a radionuclide introduced into the patient's body. PET uses a rapidly decaying material that emits positrons, sub-atomic particles that are almost immediately annihilated in collision with an electron. The result is the emission of two photons of energy that travel in almost exactly opposite directions. If both can be detected, the two events define a line through the body, which must pass through the point from which the original positron was emitted. A PET image is built up from such lines, in the same way that a CT image is built up by back-projecting detected X-rays.

One exciting new development in medical imaging is the use of these functional imaging techniques to obtain information about the behaviour of the body not at the level of gross physiological processes such as blood flow and oxygenation but at the level of the underlying biochemical reactions. We can bind, for example, the radionuclides used in PET to ligands that will attach to specific receptor cells. We can treat highly magnetic nanoparticles, which will massively enhance MRI signals, in a similar way, associating them with biological molecules that have highly specific functions. If we can identify enzymes that are found in higher concentrations in or around tumours and, for example, treat magnetic nanoparticles with ligands that bind to these enzymes, we ought to be able to generate MRI images in which even very small tumours would be clearly visible. Researchers have used this technique in an attempt to devise a highly sensitive test for breast cancer. Transferrin is a cell-surface receptor that is responsible for the sequestration of iron in mammalian cells and that is found to be 'over-expressed' in tumour cells. Treating superparamagnetic monocrystalline iron oxide nanoparticles (MIONs) with ligands for TfR massively increases the sensitivity of MRI as a test for breast tumours.

The practical application of these ideas will require the development of devices that can be produced commercially, tests that can safely and comfortably be administered to patients and the identification of clinical applications for which the tests provide an acceptable balance of sensitivity, specificity, financial cost and acceptability to patients. Finding the right niche for the test (screening, symptomatic patients, monitoring of diagnosed patients) involves a judgement about the possible contribution to a patient's case of the additional information that the test provides.

References

1. Farr RF, Allisy-Roberts PJ. *Physics for Medical Imaging*. London: W.B. Saunders, 1997.
2. Heeger DJ, Ress D. What does fMRI tell us about neuronal activity? *Nat Rev Neurosci* 2002;3:142–151.
3. Basilion JP. Breast imaging technology: current and future technologies for breast cancer. *Breast Cancer Res* 2001;3:14–16.

Problems with data

I want to introduce two complications to the account of how X-rays depict anatomical information: first, the problem of scattered photons; and second, the problem of the film's 'characteristic response'.

- *Scattered radiation.* Most photons arrive on the film after having passed through the body in a straight line. However, as shown in Figure 5.2, some of them are deflected. These scattered photons are problematic be-

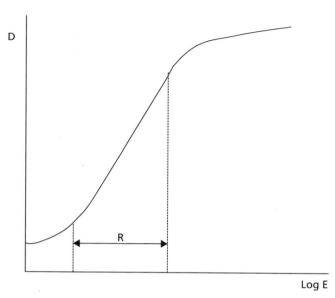

Figure 5.3 Characteristic curve of X-ray film. The plot of the amount of X-rays hitting a film (log E) against film density (D) is a straight line only over a limited range of incident radiation (R).

cause they expose a region of film which does not correspond geometrically to the region through which they passed. They contribute to the X-ray image, but they do not provide information. We say that the image data have two components: the signal, which conveys the information; and the noise, which does not. Scattered radiation is a form of noise.

- *Film response*. The X-ray works as a depiction of the anatomy because there is a direct relationship between the shade of grey on the film and a relevant property of the anatomy. This relationship exists in part because the photons hitting the film cause a chemical reaction that changes the colour of the film. Unfortunately – given the physical limitations of film – the relationship holds good only across a certain range of X-ray illumination, as shown in Figure 5.3. If the image has been taken at the wrong exposure, there may be areas of the film where the number of photons detected is too great or too small for the contrast to be an accurate reflection of the anatomy.

Information and data

What does this tell us about representation? It might be clearer if we make a distinction between data and information. In this case the image on the film provides the data. The information is what the image represents; for example, what it can tell us about the arrangement of tissues in the body. We say that the information is 'contained in' or 'carried by' the data. The data contain errors, in this case because of the scattered radiation. Information may also be missing from the data, if regions of the film are over-exposed, for example. So, to get the information we need we have to interpret the data. This might involve filtering out errors, or making inferences about missing data. The information is, in some sense, encoded in the representation and we have to decode it.

Interpreting data

Interpreting data involves adopting a perspective. I have explained how the data on an X-ray film can provide information about the X-ray-absorbent properties of the body. But we could look at the data in a different way. A physicist might use them to obtain information about the performance of the X-ray camera. A clinician might look for information in them about the presence or absence of cancer. A computer scientist interested in using computers to display images might want to work out how to create a pixel array that could serve instead of the X-ray. What counts as information is a question of perspective. This becomes clearer when we think about how to quantify the information in the image. For the clinician there might be a single piece of information: the presence or absence of cancer. For the physicist the amount of information contained in the X-ray is determined by the detail and the contrast that can be distinguished on the image. For the computer scientist the amount of disk space required to store the image is determined by the number of pixels, and the number of bytes per pixel, required to create an equivalent digital image. The clinician, the physicist and the computer scientist are all dealing with the same data, but obtaining very different information from them.

Encoded representations

We can represent the X-ray image on a computer as a pixel array, which is essentially a set of numbers. Each number has a position and a value. The number's position in the array corresponds to a location in the image and its value corresponds to the 'grey level' or brightness at that point in the image. Just as the image contains information about the anatomy, so too does the pixel array, since the image can be recreated from the array.

Fans of more recent sci-fi movies than *2001: A Space Odyssey* may recall the character in *The Matrix* who could look at streams of digits cascading down a computer screen and 'see' the people and places depicted in the software. For the rest of us, however, the information represented in a pixel array is encoded: we cannot see it by looking at the array of numbers the way we can when we look at an image. Of course, the information in an X-ray is also encoded, but the encoding is a direct consequence of the physics of the image-formation process and, because the result is an image, it is very easy to decode. We can see what the image has to show us.

Symbolic representations

The way images work as representations of information is, at first glance, very different from the way we represent information in ordinary language.

But in both cases information is encoded in the representation and has to be decoded. In language the encoding is to do with how the author's or speaker's intentions are wrapped up in what he or she writes or says. The process of decoding involves recognising the words and working out what the speaker or writer intended to convey by them. We use words as tokens, as symbols that stand for the ideas, events and objects we wish to describe, and we combine them in sentences that convey our intended meanings. The idea that we assemble representations by putting symbols into structures is a very powerful one, and later chapters will deal with it in some depth, looking both at the right symbols to use to represent clinical concepts and at how these symbols can be used to build models for different applications of health informatics. First, however, we should think about how symbolic representations can be used in computers.

Entities and relationships

Databases often represent information in terms of relationships. Relationships hold between classes of entity and we can draw up a general schema for a database by identifying the list of entities to be represented and the permitted relations between them. Building the database is then a matter of fitting the facts to be recorded into the schema. A common graphical technique for representing such schemas is the entity relationship diagram (Figure 5.4). Each class of entity is represented by a square and the squares are linked by arrows labelled with diamonds. These represent the relationships. The direction of the arrows indicates a constraint on the way entities can participate in a relationship. The example shown allows a patient to register with only one GP although a GP can have many patients registered.

The notation is not important. What matters here is the capacity to think of the world as consisting of: (1) things and (2) things that connect things. As shown in Figure 5.4, we can use entity relationship diagrams to represent facts such as patients are registered with GPs. If we were designing a database we might use this fact to determine that the database should include a relation 'registered' linking GPs and patients. You can think of this as a table with two columns, one for GPs and one for patients, and a row for each patient (Table 5.1). Note that the entity relationship diagram cannot be

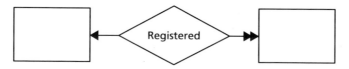

Figure 5.4 We use a square to denote an entity and an arrow labelled with a diamond to represent a relation between entities. The single head at left of the arrow with a double head at the right indicates that this is a one-to-many relation. Each patient is registered with one GP. Each GP has many patients.

Table 5.1 A database table for a binary one-to-many relation.

REGISTERED relation	
GP	Patient
Dr Dolittle	Joe Baker
Dr Dolittle	John Jones
Dr Dolitte	Mary Smith
Dr Dolots	Freida Clark
Dr Dolots	Joan Booth
Dr Dolots	Alan McKay

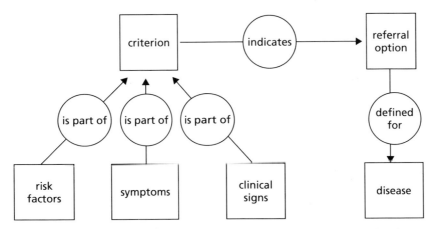

Figure 5.5 A semantic network showing how the concepts used in the referral application are related. Concepts are represented as boxes. Their relationships are represented as arrows labelled with circles.

used to represent the information that, for example, Joan Booth is registered with Dr Dolots. The formalism is designed for the representation of types, not instances of types. A looser formalism, the semantic net, can be more useful for knowledge representation. Semantic nets represent concepts and the relations between concepts and, at first glance, and indeed after a second glance, look very similar to entity relationship diagrams. An example is given in Figure 5.5. Concepts are represented as boxes; their relationships are represented as arrows labelled with circles.

Representing knowledge as relationships
Imagine that we are trying to build a knowledge base that contains information about when different categories of patients should be referred for hospital outpatient appointments. The knowledge base might be used in conjunction with a system that allows GPs to book appointments for their patients directly. Our knowledge base is intended to contain rules that have

been agreed between the hospital consultants and the GPs in an attempt to ensure that patients are referred appropriately.

What kinds of thing do we want to include in our knowledge base? We will need to make a list of the diseases that fall within the scope of the system. Let us start with the major cancers. For each one we will need to enumerate the different options for referral: e.g. urgent referral, non-urgent referral, no referral. We will also want to represent the criteria that determine which of these options is appropriate. These will be based on the patient's characteristics including not just signs and symptoms but other things such as risk factors and family circumstances.

We can approach the problem by identifying three levels at which information is to be represented. At the highest level is a model of the domain, an ontology. This specifies the kinds of thing we are dealing with: diseases, categories of referral, signs, symptoms, risk factors. It also specifies how they relate. So our ontology consists of statements such as those presented in Figure 5.6. Analysing the problem at this level we can identify the rule that patients are to be referred with specified urgency for a particular disease if all of the elements of a criterion are true, for a given patient.

The next level down consists of the sets of facts that make up the referral criteria for a disease: for example, that a 50-year-old woman with a discrete breast lump requires an urgent referral to the breast cancer clinic. These facts will make up our knowledge base. If we interpret Figure 5.6 as an entity relationship diagram, we could view it as defining a database that will be populated with these facts.

However, these facts remain general statements in the sense that they capture general truths about clinical practice rather than relate an individual patient's experience. In order to use our knowledge base to make recommendations we need to combine these general statements with case-specific facts. This is the third level.

Figure 5.6 shows a way of representing the required information at these three levels. The top level is a rule expressed in logic. We will deal with logic in Chapter 6. The point here is to note how the representation is built up as a set of relations that link the entities in the domain, and a rule that asserts that if certain relationships hold, another relationship must also hold.

Logic and probability

The general idea of health informatics is to represent clinical information, whether facts about patients or more general medical knowledge, in programs (electronic patient records, clinical information systems, etc.) that can be used to improve patient care, by guiding decision-making, for example. There are many examples of such programs, using many different forms of representation. In all of them, or pretty nearly all of them, however, the computations that are performed using those representations can be characterised, as either logical or statistical. Either the system contains logical rules that generate

Model Level: we represent a general rule which states that patients are to be referred with specified urgency for a particular disease if all of the elements of a criterion are true, for a given patient.

IF
        indicates (Criterion, Urgency, Disease)
AND
        FORALL Part (
            IF
                part_of (Criterion, Part),
            THEN
                true_for_patient (Patient, Part)
).
THEN
        refer_with_urgency (Patient, Disease, Urgency)

Application Level: each criterion has one or more parts that must all be true if a patient is to be referred.

indicates(criterion1, urgent_referral, breast_cancer)

part_of(criterion1, has_breast_lump)
part_of(criterion1, over_50)

Patient Data: we must represent the facts that are referred to in the criteria.

true_for_patient (joan, has_breast_lump).
true_for_patient (joan, over_50).

Figure 5.6 A logical representation of the knowledge required for a referrals application.

advice on the basis of the information represented or it makes inferences from calculations based on numerical data. Chapter 6 considers the theoretical background to the first of these approaches: logic.

References

1. Cycorp. *What is Cyc?* http://www.cyc.com/cyc/technology/whatiscyc (accessed 12 February 2004).
2. Searle, J. Minds, brains, and programs. *Behav Brain Sci* 1980;3:417–424.

CHAPTER 6
Logic

Logic is the study of arguments[1]. An argument is a connected series of statements intended to establish a conclusion. It consists of a set of premises and a conclusion. In assessing arguments, we have to consider two properties: truth and validity. Truth is a property of statements: some statements are true and some are not. A statement is true if it describes something that is the case. This is so obvious that it is odd to hear it stated. Validity is an equally straightforward, but less familiar, concept. Validity is a property of arguments. We say that an argument is valid if the conclusion follows from the premises. More precisely, we say that an argument is valid if the truth of the premises guarantees the truth of the conclusion. The important point here is that truth and validity are different concepts. We can make a judgement about the validity of an argument without making a judgement about the truth of its premises.

Logicians developed formal languages to be used in the analysis of arguments and these languages are, in effect, the forerunners of computer languages, which means that an understanding of logic is a prerequisite for an understanding of topics in computer science as diverse as databases, algorithms and decision-making. (A familiarity with logic is also an important aid to clear and analytical thinking, which is an exceptionally useful skill in a field such as this one.)

Propositional calculus

The simplest form of logic is known as the propositional calculus. A proposition is any sentence that can be true or false. So, for example, 'Manchester is the capital of England' is a proposition while 'yar boo sucks' is not. True and false are the two possible truth values in the propositional calculus. The propositional calculus provides a set of rules for building up complex propositions from simple propositions and also a set of rules for drawing inferences from propositions.

The rules for how complex propositions are built up involve what are known as operators. There are four operators: *and, or, implies* and *not*. The first three are used to link propositions; the fourth is a prefix. Propositions are often represented with letters, so let us say, in this case, that *p* and *q* are propositions. We can then say that *p and q*, *p or q* and *p implies q* are also propositions. So are *not p* and *not q*. And so too is (*p or q*) *implies* (*p or not* (*q and p*)), to give a more complex example.

The truth of the compound propositions is determined by the truth or otherwise of their elements. If *p* is true then *not p* is false, if *p* is true and *q* is true then *p and q* is true, if either *p* is true or *q* is true then *p or q* is true. All of this should seem intuitive, since these rules capture what we usually mean by the words 'not', 'and' and 'or'.

The rule for implication, however, can cause confusion. If *p* is true and *q* is true then *p implies q* is true. This should be clear enough. If *p* is true and *q* is false then *p implies q* is false. This too should correspond to what we normally understand by the word 'implies'. If *p* is false, however, then *p implies q* is true whether or not *q* is true. Ian Hislop, the editor of *Private Eye* and target of numerous libel suits once emerged from court to say, 'if this is justice then I am a banana'. The point is that if a premise (this is justice) is false then anything can be concluded from it, even something completely ridiculous (I am a banana). I will not pretend that this is not confusing but, fortunately, it is not a form of argument encountered very often.

Truth tables

To see how these rules work in practice we can draw up what is called a 'truth table'. In a truth table each component proposition and each step in the construction of the final proposition has a column. There is a row for each possible combination of truth values, and so a table for two propositions has four rows, for three propositions eight, for four propositions sixteen and so on. We say that each row corresponds to an interpretation of the complex propositions. It corresponds to a possible set of circumstances. Consider Table 6.1. The first two columns give the four possible combinations of truth values for *p* and *q* and the remaining four columns give the truth values of the complex propositions built up from *p* and *q*.

Entailment

So, we have a definition of propositions, a set of operators for composing complex propositions and a set of rules that explain how the truth of complex propositions is determined by the truth of their component propositions. The final element in the propositional calculus is a method for establishing when an argument or an inference is valid. A valid inference is one where if the premises are true, the conclusion must be true. We normally set out

Table 6.1 Truth tables for the propositions: *not p, not p or q, p implies q* and (*p and (p implies q)*).

p	q	not p	not p or q	p implies q	p and (p implies q)
T	T	F	T	T	T
T	F	F	F	F	F
F	T	T	T	T	F
F	F	T	T	T	F

arguments as follows, with the set of premises above and the conclusion below a horizontal line:

p implies q

p

———————

q

We can establish validity in two ways: by looking at all the possible interpretations of the arguments, i.e. at the truth tables; or by applying syntactic rules in order to arrive at the conclusion from the premises. These two approaches deal with *semantic* and *syntactic* entailment, respectively.

If we take a set of propositions S and a proposition P, we can say that the set S semantically entails P if for every interpretation in which S is true, P is true. If we look at Table 6.1, we see that for every row in which the set of propositions {*p*, (*p implies q*)} is true, *q* is also true. We can therefore say that the set of propositions {*p*, (*p implies q*)} semantically entails *q*. The argument above is valid.

Of course, in the case of any example sufficiently complex for it to be necessary to test the inference, to use truth tables to establish semantic entailment would be horrendously unwieldy. Syntactic entailment is a much more useful method. It consists of a set of steps. There are two kinds of step, the application of 'rules of inference' and the application of 'rewrite rules'. Rules of inference allow us to add new propositions to the set of propositions known to be valid. Rewrite rules allow us to restate propositions in different forms. Both sets of rules can be seen to be valid by checking the truth tables. Syntactic entailment is, in other words, grounded in semantic entailment.

Rules of inference

There are nine rules of inference, shown in Table 6.2. The best known, Modus Ponens, is that given a set of propositions which includes the propositions *p* and *p implies q*, we can add *q* to the set. Take a moment or two to check that all the rules in Table 6.2 seem to make sense, in other words, that the conclusions (the propositions below the line) are clearly semantically entailed by the premises (the propositions above the line).

Logical equivalence and rewrite rules

The meaning of the operators in the propositional calculus is defined by truth tables. If we look at the fourth and fifth columns in Table 6.1, we can see that *p implies q* has the same truth table as *not p or q*. This means that wherever *p implies q* appears, we can rewrite it as *not p or q*, and vice versa. Logically the two statements are indistinguishable. We call such pairs of statements 'logical equivalences'. Some well-known equivalences are used in syntactic entailment as 'rewrite rules', since they can allow propositions to be restated in a form that makes it possible to apply the rules of inference to establish that an

Table 6.2 The rules of inference.

p implies q	*p implies q*	*p implies q*
p	*not q*	*q implies r*
———	———	———
q	*not p*	*p implies r*
1 Modus Ponens	**2 Modus Tollens**	**3 Hypothetical syllogism**
p or q		*(p implies q) and (r implies s)*
not p	*p and q*	*p or r*
———	———	———
q	*p*	*q or s*
4 Disjunctive syllogism	**5 Simplification**	**6 Constructive dilemma**
p		
q	*p implies q*	*p*
———	———	———
p and q	*p implies (p and q)*	*p or q*
7 Conjunction	**8 Absorption**	**9 Disjunction**

inference does indeed follow from a set of premises. A list of well-known rules is given in Table 6.3.

Using the propositional calculus

Here is one example of the way the propositional calculus can be used in medical reasoning, taken from the classic Ledley and Lusted paper on the foundations of medical diagnosis.[2]

A five-week-old infant was observed by the mother to have progressive difficulty in breathing during a five-day period. No respiratory problem had been observed after birth. Physical examination showed a well-nourished infant with haemangiomas (blood vessel tumours) on the lower neck, left ear and lower lip. The physician decided that one of three abnormalities

Table 6.3 Thirteen logical equivalences used as rewrite rules.

   i. *not (p and q) = (not p) or (not q)*
  ii. *not (p or q) = (not p) and (not q)*
 iii. *p and q = q and p*
 iv. *p or q = q or p*
  v. *p and (q and r) = (p and q) and r*
 vi. *p or (q or r) = (p or q) or r*
 vii. *p or (q and r) = (p or q) and (p or r)*
viii. *p and (q or r) = (p and q) or (p and r)*
 ix. *p = not not p*
  x. *p implies q = (not p) implies (not q)*
 xi. *p implies q = (not p) or q*
 xii. *(p and q) implies r = p implies (q implies r)*
xiii. *p implies (q and r) = (p implies q) and (p implies r)*

might be causing the respiratory distress: a prominent thymus gland, a deep haemangioma in mediastinum or a dermoid cyst in the mediastinum. An X-ray examination was ordered.

Given the following three pieces of medical knowledge, show that a negative X-ray would confirm, for each of the three diseases, whether or not the patient had that disease.

1 If the patient did not have a deep haemangioma, then haemangiomas would not be visible on the surface.
2 If the patient did not have a prominent thymus gland but did have a deep haemangioma and a dermoid cyst, then a mass would be visible on the X-ray.
3 A patient with a prominent thymus gland and either a deep haemangioma or a dermoid cyst in the mediastinum would have respiratory problems and would have a mass visible on the X-ray.

Let us give each of the diseases and each of the symptoms a label:
   D1 = a prominent thymus gland
   D2 = a deep haemangioma in mediastinum
   D3 = a dermoid cyst in the mediastinum

   S1 = respiratory distress
   S2 = visible haemangioma
   S3 = mass visible on X-ray

The next step is to represent each of the three facts using the propositional calculus:
   1 *not* D2 *implies* (*not* S2)
   2 *not* D1 *and* D2 *and* D3 *implies* S3
   3 D1 *and* (D2 *or* D3) *implies* (S1 *and* S3)
We add to these facts the two bits of clinical information that we have:
   4 S1
   5 S2
and the thing that we are hypothesising:
   6 *not* S3
which gives us our set of facts. We want to infer, for each of D1, D2 and D3 either the proposition or its negation. Well, we can infer D2 straightaway from propositions 1 and 5, using Modus Tollens to infer *not* (*not* D2), which can be rewritten as D2. So let us add D2 to the set of facts as proposition 7:
   7 D2.
The best strategy for inferring something about D1 would seem to be to look at proposition 3, and a useful first step here might be to separate out the two terms in the conclusion. We can rewrite 3 to give us D1 *and* (D2 *or* D3) *implies* S1 and D1 *and* (D2 *or* D3) *implies* S3 and then apply the simplification rule to get:
   8 D1 *and* (D2 *or* D3) *implies* S3
from which we can infer:
   9 *not* [D1 *and* (D2 *or* D3)]

using Modus Tollens and proposition 6. This may not look immediately useful but rewriting it with equivalences i, ii and vii (from Table 6.3) gives us *not* D1 *or not* D2 and *not* D1 *or not* D3, from which we can infer:

   10 *not* D1 *or not* D2

using the simplification rule. This can be used with 7 to make a disjunctive syllogism, which allows us to infer:

   11 *not* D1.

We can use Modus Tollens again to infer *not* (*not* D1 *and* D2 *and* D3) from 2 and 6. Rewriting this we get:

   12 D1 *or not* D2 *or not* D3.

Again, using the disjunctive syllogism with 7 and 11 we can infer:

   13 *not* D3.

We can say therefore that if the infant has a negative X-ray, we can confirm that he or she is suffering from a deep haemangioma in mediastinum and not a prominent thymus gland or a dermoid cyst.

Proof by resolution

We used the rule for disjunctive syllogism in a number of steps in the above example. This rule is the basis for another technique for testing inferences, a technique known as proof by resolution. This technique is worth mentioning here because it can be mechanised and so is the basis for most attempts to program computers to prove theorems[3]. The first step is to convert each statement into what is called normal form, by rewriting it using logical equivalences, such as the one discussed between *p implies q* and *not p or q*. Any proposition can be converted into normal form. In normal form, all propositions are disjunctions of negated or not negated simple propositions. The *implies* or *and* operators are not used and the *not* operator occurs only within the tightest brackets. Anyone interested in such puzzles may like to check that the three rules above can be rewritten as follows:

   1 D2 *or not* S2
   2 D1 *or not* D2 *or not* D3 *or* S3
   3 i   *not* D1 *or not* D2 *or* S1
      ii *not* D1 *or not* D3 *or* S1
      iii *not* D1 *or not* D2 *or* S3
      iv *not* D1 *or not* D3 *or* S3

We add to these facts the two bits of clinical information that we have:

   4 S1
   5 S2

and our hypothesis:

   6 *not* S3.

The way proof by resolution works is in essence by applying the rule for disjunctive syllogism. Whenever we have a fact *p*, we can remove all mentions of *not p* from a disjunction. Given the observations in 4 and 5 we can remove all mentions of *not* S1 and of *not* S2 from rules 1–3. Equally, given observation 6, we can remove all mentions of S3:

   1 D2
   2 D1 *or not* D2 *or not* D3
   3 i   *not* D1 *or not* D2 *or* S1
     ii   *not* D1 *or not* D3 *or* S1
    iii   *not* D1 *or not* D2
    iv   *not* D1 *or not* D3

Our first rule now allows us to infer D2. So we can remove all mentions of *not* D2 from all the other rules.

   1 D2
   2 D1 *or not* D3
   3 i   *not* D1 *or* S1
     ii   *not* D1 *or not* D3 *or* S1
    iii   *not* D1
    iv   *not* D1 *or not* D3

Rule 3iii now allows us to infer *not* D1. A final step 'resolving' D1 and *not* D1 allows us to infer *not* D3 from rule 2. Problem solved. A positive X-ray confirms a deep haemangioma in mediastinum and excludes both a prominent thymus gland and a dermoid cyst in the mediastinum.

    This reasoning process is completely mechanical and can be programmed fairly simply. It is clearly unnecessary to program a computer to solve such a simple problem but when there are very large databases of facts to be considered, such a program could be useful. To make these programs work, however, requires a more sophisticated approach than in this example to the representation of relevant knowledge. The rest of this chapter explores some such approaches.

Predicate calculus

In practice, the propositional calculus is too crude a tool for most automated reasoning applications. Consider the following rule: if A is the father of B and B is the father of C, then A is the grandfather of C. To express this in the propositional calculus we would have to have three propositions:

   P1: A is the father of B
   P2: B is the father of C
   P3: A is the grandfather of C

And a rule:

   P1 *and* P2 *implies* P3.

But we cannot use this to work out who is or is not a grandfather on the basis of a set of facts about who is a father of whom. For that we need a formalism capable of revealing how statements work as statements about things. We need to look inside the propositions. Predicate calculus provides exactly that.

    A predicate can be a bit like an adjective, a way of expressing that some thing or class of things has a particular property. It can also be a way of expressing a relation that exists between two or more things or classes of thing. Consider the following statement in predicate calculus:

For all A, B, C: father (A, B) *and* father (B, C) *implies* grandfather (A, C).

The letters A, B and C are variables, place-holders for examples of the class of thing we are talking about (people, men, male members of the family – whatever the group under discussion happens to be). The words that precede the parentheses are the predicates asserted of the combination of variables. They represent relationships that hold for some of the individuals in the domain of interest. This all sounds a bit mathematical, but by simply looking at the statement you can see how it expresses the meaning of grandfather. The statement consists of three predicates linked by operators of the same kind that we saw in the propositional calculus. The only other element to the predicate calculus is what are called 'quantifiers'.

Quantification

Any statement in the predicate calculus can be either universally quantified or existentially quantified. A universally quantified statement about class X is true for all examples of X. The rule for the definition of grandfather is an example of this. An existentially quantified statement about X is true for at least one example of X. Existentially quantified statements can, however, always be converted into universally quantified statements. There is a simple logical equivalence such that a statement of the form 'predicate A is true for an example of X' is equivalent to 'it is not true that predicate A is not true for all X'. If we say that some breast cancers are inoperable, in other words, this is logically equivalent to saying that it is not the case that no breast cancer is inoperable.

Using the predicate calculus

Consider the following guideline for the urgent referral of a child with a headache:

Headache of recent origin with one or more of the following features:
* increasing in severity or frequency
* noted to be worse in the morning or causing early wakening
* associated with vomiting
* associated with neurological signs (e.g. squint, ataxia)
* associated with behavioural change or deterioration in school performance

We can represent this rule in the predicate calculus using a general rule about the referral of patients suffering from particular kinds of headaches together with a set of facts about the features of headache that suggest referral is necessary.

For all Pa, S, Pr and V:
   patient_has_symptom (Pa, S) *and*
   symptom_is_kind_of (S, headache) *and*
   symptom_has_feature (S, Pr, V) *and*
   symptom_feature_indicates_referral (headache, Pr, V) *implies*

patient_should_be_referred (Pa)

symptom_feature_indicates_referral (headache, severity, increasing)
symptom_feature_indicates_referral (headache, frequency, increasing)
symptom_feature_indicates_referral (headache, diurnal_variation,
   worse_in_morning)
symptom_feature_indicates_referral (headache, associated_with,
   vomiting)
symptom_feature_indicates_referral (headache, associated_with,
   neurological signs)
symptom_feature_indicates_referral (headache, associated_with,
   behavioural_change)

We can imagine how this rule could be interpreted in a computer program used to identify whether there are grounds for referring a patient. The rule uses five predicates. The predicate in the conclusion asserts a particular property of the patient, that he or she should be referred. The first predicate **patient_has_symptom** would be used to retrieve all the recorded symptoms from the patient record. Our computer program could retrieve them all at once or one at a time. In a real system, an additional check would be needed to ensure that only current symptoms are selected. The symptoms would then be tested using rules about terminology in order to identify the ones that were headaches or kinds of headaches, using the predicate **symptom_is_kind_of.** The next predicate **symptom_has_feature** would be used to retrieve further information about the symptoms, in terms of their listed properties and values. These would then be tested against the facts used to represent the specific features of headache that suggest referral. These are represented in the predicate **symptom_feature_indicates_referral.** The program might terminate when it has found a match, which would be sufficient ground to suggest referral, or it might identify all the possible grounds. Since the rule is universally quantified, we know that any combination of Pa, S, Pr and V for which the first four predicates are true is a ground for referral.

The difficult element in all this is the last matching step: testing the features of headaches against the criteria. How can we be sure that the terms in which the patient history is recorded match those used in the rule? Writing the rules in logic is the easy bit; the hard part is sorting out the terms used to instantiate the variables. We could provide a set of drop-down menus with predefined terms, so that *headache* would appear with a pick-list of terms such as *worse_in_morning* and *associated_with_vomiting.* There are disadvantages to such menus, however. The alternative is to rely on the software to map from what the doctor writes, 'headaches, nauseous', for example, to the terms used in the set of facts.

In practice we have to constrain how the history is recorded. It is important to minimise the problems associated with that constraint: we have to design better and simpler user interfaces so that records can be created from standard sets of terms. We also need to work out how best to build sets of terms that allow doctors to express exactly what they want to say about their patients' headaches while still using words that can serve as symbols in logical rules. In the mean time the users of clinical systems must decide how far they are prepared to use standard terms, such as the Read Codes, in order to achieve the benefits associated with systems that incorporate this kind of decision support.

Relations and normal form

Before we leave this example, we should think a little more about how we represent information in predicates. A predicate is a relation and a set of statements, such as the six statements of *symptom_feature_indicates_referral* above, defines a relation. There are certain principles we should follow when we try and work out which relations make up the best representation of a domain. Some of these principles are known to people who create relational databases, as the rules that define the First, Second, Third, Fourth and Fifth levels of Normal Form[4]. (This is a different notion of normal form to that introduced in the section on Resolution.) Let us look again at the set of facts we need to be able to represent about the patient. First, we need to have a predicate *patient_has_symptom* and to assert a statement (or clause) of the predicate to state that the patient has a headache:

patient_has_symptom ('fred smith', headache)

But, as we have seen, we need to be able to say something more about the headache. One way would be to replace this statement with a more precise one:

patient_has_symptom ('fred smith', severe_headache)

But this is clearly unworkable if the term to be used for the symptom has to capture a long and complex description:

patient_has_symptom ('fred smith', severe_headaches_of_increasing_ frequency worse_in_morning_and_associated_with_vomiting)

Instead it might be better to include one term for headache and add other terms that capture the description. We could do this by extending our relation from being a binary one (between patient and symptom) to one that covers many more variables.

patient_has_symptom ('fred smith', headache, severe, increasing_ frequency, worse_in_morning, associated_with_vomiting)

This, however, is problematic. If we design rules to be used in conjunction with these facts, we need to know how many variables appear in the relation. This is the idea behind 'First Normal Form' in database theory. A relational database is in First Normal Form if all the occurrences of a record type contain the same number of fields. In logic we say that a predicate consists of a set of statements each with the same number of fields (although in logic we generally use the term 'argument' or 'parameter' rather than 'field'). So we could put each element of the description of the headache into a separate statement, within a relation having three arguments:

patient_has_symptom ('fred smith', headache, severe)
patient_has_symptom ('fred smith', headache, increasing_frequency)
patient_has_symptom ('fred smith', headache, worse_in_morning)
patient_has_symptom ('fred smith', headache, associated_with_vomiting)

This, however, is inefficient, since we are repeating **'fred smith'** unnecessarily. In terms of database theory, this relation violates Second Normal Form, because the attribute in the third argument is not, formally speaking, an attribute of Fred Smith but of his headache. The appropriate representation is therefore:

patient_has_symptom ('fred smith', headache)
symptom_has_feature (headache, severe)
symptom_has_feature (headache, increasing_frequency)
symptom_has_feature (headache, worse_in_morning)
symptom_has_feature (headache, associated_with_vomiting)

We could break the representation down even further. This version conceals some structure in some of the terms used to describe the headache. For example, the term *increasing_frequency* might be viewed not as a description of the headache but as a description of a property of the headache (its frequency). It would be better to separate terms for the properties of the headache **(severity, frequency,** etc.) from terms that describe those properties **(increasing, worse_in_morning,** etc.).

symptom_has_feature (headache, severity, increasing)
symptom_has_feature (headache, frequency, increasing)
symptom_has_feature (headache, diurnal_variation, worse_in_morning)
symptom_has_feature (headache, associated_with, vomiting)
symptom_has_feature (headache, associated_with, neurological_signs)
symptom_has_feature (headache, associated_with, behavioural_change)

One of the difficulties with this example is that having broken up the description of the headache into several distinct statements, we no longer have any way of knowing whether the statements are all descriptions of the same headache. A patient's record might contain statements about several headaches. We need a new term that will uniquely identify the particular headache we are interested in. The best thing to do is to generate a unique identifier for the symptom, let us call it **symxxx1**, and include the statement that **symxxx1** is a headache.

patient_has_symptom ('fred smith', symxxx1)

symptom_is_kind_of (symxxx1, headache)

symptom_has_feature (symxxx1, severity, increasing)
symptom_has_feature (symxxx1, frequency, increasing)
symptom_has_feature (symxxx1, diurnal_variation, worse_in_morning)
symptom_has_feature (symxxx1, associated_with, vomiting)

symptom_has_feature (symxxx1, associated_with, neurological_signs)
symptom_has_feature (symxxx1, associated_with, behavioural_change)

This is the representation assumed in the example in the previous section. It does not include everything one would want, by any means. The statements would need to be associated with lots of additional information, such as dates, and who recorded the statements and so on. It is, however, a fairly clear and robust presentation of the information required for a realistic piece of clinical reasoning.

Fuzzy logic

True and false are the two possible truth values in conventional logic. We sometimes represent them with numbers, so true = 1 and false = 0. What would happen if, instead of forcing everything to be either true or false, we allowed truth values to take any intermediate value between 0 and 1?

Fuzzy logic is a variant of logic, based on fuzzy set theory[5]. In classical set theory, an object is either a member of a set or it is not. One way of defining a set is to compute a 'membership function' for the set. If you had, in classic set theory, a set of patients with fever, and you drew a graph of the patients' temperature against the value of the membership function, it would look like the first graph in Figure 6.1. Patients with temperatures up to a certain threshold would have a value of 0 for the membership function. Above the threshold the value would be 1. The threshold defines the set of fevered patients. In fuzzy set theory we allow membership functions to behave like

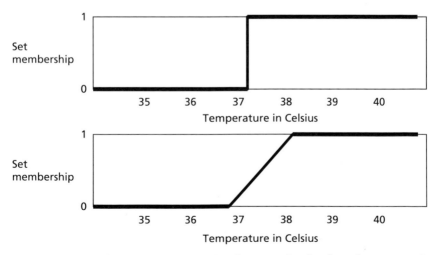

Figure 6.1 Two graphs showing membership functions for the class of patients with fever. The first defines a traditional 'crisp' set; the second, a 'fuzzy' set in which some members are allowed to be partly members of the set.

the second graph in Figure 6.1. There are people who have fever and people who do not have fever, but there is a grey area between the two.

We can define fuzzy equivalents of the standard operations on sets: complement, intersection, union and subsumption. If a fuzzy set A has a membership function m(A), the complement of A is a fuzzy set defined by the membership function 1 − m(A). We say fuzzy set A is a subset of fuzzy set B if all members of A have an equal or higher membership value for B than they do for A. If two fuzzy sets A and B have membership functions m(A) and n(B), the intersection is a fuzzy set defined by the function that always takes the lower of the membership values given by the two functions. The union of the two fuzzy sets is the fuzzy set with a membership function that is the higher of the two. Consider an application of fuzzy logic in the management of ICU patients using the fuzzy sets whose membership functions are shown in Figure 6.2[6]. Three fuzzy sets are defined for a patient's

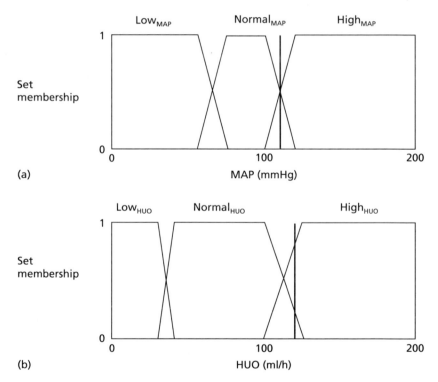

Figure 6.2 (a) Membership functions of three fuzzy sets for mean arterial blood pressure (MAP). The bold vertical line is drawn at an MAP of 110 mmHg, where the membership values for the three sets are 0 (Low$_{MAP}$), 0.5 (Normal$_{MAP}$) and 0.5 (High$_{MAP}$), respectively. (b) Membership functions of three fuzzy sets for hourly urine output (HUO). The bold vertical line is drawn at an HUO of 110 ml/h, where the membership values for the three sets are 0 (Low$_{HUO}$), 0.2 (Normal$_{HUO}$) and 0.8 (High$_{HUO}$), respectively. From [6] with permission. © 2003 American Thoracic Society.

mean arterial pressure (MAP): Low$_{MAP}$, Normal$_{MAP}$ and High$_{MAP}$, so that a patient with an MAP of 110 mmHg is given a value of 0 for the membership function of Low$_{MAP}$ but 0.5 for both Normal$_{MAP}$ and High$_{MAP}$. Let us say that our patient also has fairly high hourly urine output (HUO), and hence a value of 0 for the membership function of the set Low$_{HUO}$ and 0.2 for Normal$_{HUO}$ but 0.8 for High$_{HUO}$. If we combine the sets High$_{MAP}$ and High$_{HUO}$, our patient will have a membership value of 0.5 for the intersection High$_{MAP}$ and High$_{HUO}$ and a membership value of 0.8 for the union High$_{MAP}$ and High$_{HUO}$.

The *complement*, *union* and *intersection* operations play the roles for set theory that the operators *not*, *or* and *and* play in logic. We can use them to construct complicated fuzzy conditions. These conditions can form the antecedents in a process of reasoning. The next question, then, is how do we do fuzzy reasoning? What happens to fuzzy truth values when we infer conclusions from antecedents? One approach to reasoning is to say that the conclusion of an argument should have a truth value no greater than that of the antecedent. Say we have a rule in the ICU that the intravenous fluid rate (IFR) should be low for patients with high blood pressure and high HUO. Assume we have membership functions, as shown in Figure 6.3, for five different settings of IFR. The output of this rule for our patient will be a modified version of the membership function for the fuzzy set Low$_{IFR}$, truncated so that its truth value cannot be greater than 0.5, since 0.5 is the truth value our patient has for the antecedent of the rule: High$_{MAP}$ *and* High$_{HUO}$.

Fuzzy logic is often used in applications where some output value (e.g. IFR) has to be computed on the basis of a given set of input values. In a typical application there would be a set of rules, like the one above, each saying which fuzzy set of output values should be used for a given combination of

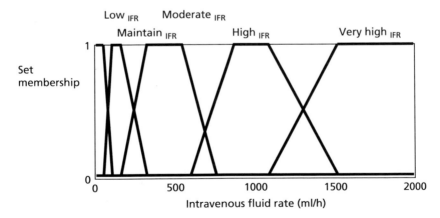

Figure 6.3 Graphs showing membership functions for the fuzzy sets used in an ICU application to control intravenous fluid rate (IFR). From [6] with permission. © 2003 American Thoracic Society.

fuzzy sets of input values. To determine the exact output value to be used for a specific combination of input values, all the rules have to be evaluated. To go back to the patient above, we know the MAP and the HUO, so we know the membership values for each of the fuzzy sets Low_{MAP}, $Normal_{MAP}$, $High_{MAP}$, Low_{HUO}, $Normal_{HUO}$ and $High_{HUO}$. Each of the nine possible combinations would be associated with a rule to be evaluated, resulting in nine modifications of the output membership functions, as shown in Table 6.4. These modified output functions must then be aggregated. One approach to aggregation is to create a new membership function that is the maximum of the values for each of the nine. Of course, five of the nine rule outputs in our example are functions that are truncated to 0 because our patient has a membership value of 0 for Low_{HUO} and Low_{MAP}. The final step in the process is to derive a precise output value from the aggregated membership function. We need to set the IFR to a specific value. One way of doing this is to calculate the centroid of the aggregated output function (the mean of the values under the curve).

Fuzzy logic has proved enormously successful as an approach to building control systems for fairly simple systems such as washing machines and microwave ovens. It is still in its infancy as a tool in clinical applications but it could be a powerful technique for capturing intuitions about how systems should respond to roughly defined categories.

Conclusion

This chapter has introduced three of the best-known forms of logic. The simplest, propositional calculus, is sufficient to explain how logic works as a mechanical process for the derivation of valid inferences from premises. The second, predicate calculus, serves to introduce ideas about knowledge representation, about how the use of logic in practical problems requires careful thought about the structure of the relations employed to express the facts used in logical reasoning. The third, fuzzy logic, gives some idea about how non-standard logic can be used in tasks with particular demands, such as the representation of imprecise information. Chapters 7, 8 and 9 look in more detail at issues of

Table 6.4 The intravenous fluid rate (IFR) is determined by a combination of mean arterial pressure (MAP) and hourly urine output (HUO). There are three fuzzy sets for ranges of values of MAP and three for HUO, hence nine combinations. Each combination is associated with one of the five fuzzy sets for ranges of values of IFR.

	MAP		
HUO	*low*	*normal*	*high*
low	very high	moderate	low
normal	high	maintain	low
high	moderate	maintain	low

knowledge representation. The representation of uncertainty is returned to at the end of this part in Chapters 10 and 11, which deal with probability.

References

1. Priest G. *Logic: A Very Short Introduction*. Oxford: Oxford University Press, 2000.
2. Ledley RS, Lusted LB. Reasoning foundations of medical diagnosis. *Science* 1959;130:9–21.
3. Kowalski R. *Logic for Problem Solving*. Amsterdam: North-Holland; 1979 (this book is now out of print but available online at http://www-lp.doc.ic.ac.uk/UserPages/ staff/ rak/rak.html).
4. Brookshear JG. *Computer Science: An Overview*, 6th edn. Reading, MA: Addison-Wesley, 2000.
5. Krause P, Clark D. *Representing Uncertain Information: An Artificial Intelligence Approach*. Oxford: Intellect Books, 1979.
6. Bates JH, Young MP. Applying fuzzy logic to medical decision making in the intensive care unit. *Am J Respir Crit Care Med* 2003;167(7):948–952.

CHAPTER 7
Clinical terms

In Chapter 5 we looked at the concept of representation and considered how words are used as symbols to convey meaning. I said then that later chapters would look in detail at how to choose the right symbols and how to put them together into structures that would serve as representations. This is the first of three chapters on that topic. My father is a chemist and my mental picture of these structured representations is rather like those molecular models in which coloured balls representing atoms are held together by plastic struts representing chemical bonds. Here the balls represent the basic underlying concepts in the domain and the plastic struts, the relationships that hold between them.

Chapter 6 introduced the idea of using relationships between concepts as a way of representing facts about a domain, in the discussion of predicate logic and its applications. This chapter looks at clinical terminology and considers a number of different attempts to define a controlled vocabulary of clinical concepts. The focus here is more on the terms that are used and less on the facts that one might want to represent about them; about the name used for a disease or for a treatment, rather than about how to represent the fact that this disease is treated using that drug; more about the coloured balls than the plastic struts. However, as the approaches we shall consider grow in sophistication, it will become apparent that they are less and less lists of terms and more and more mechanisms by which complex concepts are represented by specifying relationships between sets of symbols.

Redundancy and ambiguity

Consider the following list of words: *tumour, neoplasm, carcinoma, cancer, malignancy, lump, abnormal growth, mass, proliferative disease*. These are all words that could be used to describe what was wrong with a patient suffering with a particular form of cancer. The words all share a certain commonality of meaning. They are not exact synonyms, however. Some are quite general terms that refer to the central symptom of the disease – a lump or mass – without necessarily carrying any implications for diagnosis. There are also differences between the diagnostic terms: *carcinoma* is a more precise diagnosis than *cancer*.

These differences in precision and emphasis occur in medical language because they are features of language in general. We are able to communicate effectively using natural language because we bring to bear enormous amounts of background knowledge and an understanding of the context when we interpret the words that make up a sentence. Many of the communication problems in health care occur when the people involved do not share the same background. Problems also arise when words are used in computer software without an appropriate context, for example, as labels that define categories. It is increasingly important for computerised patient record systems to be able to identify all the patients with a particular condition, say diabetes. Simply searching the records for any occurrence of the word would probably succeed on most occasions but fail on many others. Consider a search using the word 'diabetes'. This would only detect patients whose diagnosis was recorded using this precise word. It would not detect patients who were recorded as 'diabetic' or 'NIDDM' (a common abbreviation for 'non-insulin-dependent diabetes mellitus'). It would, however, include patients whose records contained the words in other contexts, for example, 'suspected diabetes' or 'worried about diabetes' or 'son has diabetes'.

Standard clinical terminologies

Controlled clinical terminologies, or coding systems, have been developed in attempt to solve these problems. A controlled clinical terminology is sometimes said to 'define' a standard set of terms; by this it is meant that it provides a list of all the terms that are considered to be within the standard. It is generally not the case that the terminology provides a 'definition' of each of the terms in the standard, in the sense of providing a strict set of rules that explain how the terms are to be used. Controlled terminologies, therefore, should be viewed as attempts to solve the terminological problems caused by the use of confusing or non-standard terms and by the plethora of synonyms, not necessarily as attempts to impose rigid definitions of what terms mean or precise criteria for how they should be applied, although some terminologies do provide definitions for the concepts for which they provide codes.

The issue of terminology is often confused with that of coding. Many terminologies associate an alphanumeric code with each term that falls within the standard. So, for example, one of the terminologies discussed later in this chapter is known as the Read Codes. This includes a concept, *malignant tumour of breast*, which has a code X78WM. What is the advantage of the five-character code? Many people assume that somehow the code has a meaning for computer systems. Not really. All that the computer system requires of a terminology is that all cases of breast cancer are identified with some unique label. For its purposes *malignant tumour of breast* is as good a label as X78WM. Except that, of course it takes more memory to store a 26-character string than a five-character code, and, as some readers may remember, disk space and random access memory (RAM) used to be expensive enough to make it worth worrying about such things. That is not so much of an issue now. It could, however, be argued that there is still an advantage in using codes. The argument would be that if the character string is simply serving as a label for the concept, it is better to have a label that looks like a label, i.e. one that obviously has no other meaning, rather than one which looks like an ordinary sentence. It can be helpful to associate each concept with a set of possible linguistic descriptors, either the various English synonyms for a disease or, for systems with international application, terms in different languages. Where this is done, it helps to make a clear distinction between the unique identifier of the concept and the various text strings that different applications might associate with it.

How do you go about creating a complete set of terms for use in, for example, recording encounters in general practice? One strategy would be to try and identify the different categories of terms that are used: history/symptoms, examination/signs, diagnostic procedures, laboratory procedures, etc. Within each category one might identify subcategories and subcategories of subcategories, so that the whole thing expands like a family tree. Medicine seems well suited to such a hierarchical decomposition and most, if not all, terminologies work this way. In the rest of this chapter, four are considered: ICD-10, MeSH terms, the Read Codes and SNOMED CT.

ICD-10

The International Classification of Diseases (ICD) is an initiative sponsored by the WHO to produce a standard set of terms for use in recording public health statistics[1]. The scheme developed out of work done by nineteenth-century statisticians such as William Farr and Jacques Bertillon, who were primarily interested in causes of death. The standardisation of the recording of causes of death is still a major focus for the ICD, although the current standard has been expanded to allow the recording of diseases and related information. Indeed, as early as 1860, Florence Nightingale was calling for Farr's scheme to be adapted to allow the tabulation of hospital morbidity.

Farr based his classification on five categories: epidemic diseases, constitutional diseases, local diseases (arranged by anatomical site), developmental diseases and diseases that are the direct result of injury. The current, tenth, revision (ICD-10) retains the same essential shape in that diseases are classified anatomically, except where it is more convenient to group them on some other basis.

The ICD system of classification is associated with a number of ancillary classifications, as shown in Figure 7.1. There are various speciality-specific subsystems and also other classifications, covering topics such as disability. Within ICD-10 itself there are three elements: the core three-character codes; the fourth character specialisations and a set of tabulated lists, which are short summaries of certain codes covering specific categories of mortality.

The core of ICD-10 is the set of three-character codes for each and every disease, cause of injury or related condition that falls within the standard. When you buy ICD-10, what you buy is in effect a long list of

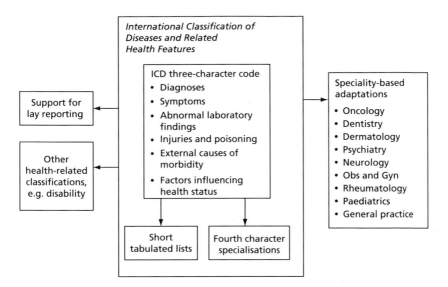

Figure 7.1 An overview of the International Classification of Diseases.

such three-character codes and their associated definitions. The list is divided into 21 chapters, as shown in Table 7.1. Each chapter covers an anatomical area or a class of diseases or related information. Each chapter is assigned a set of codes. Within the chapters, codes are divided into blocks; so, for example, in Chapter II, on neoplasms, codes C00–C75 correspond to malignant neoplasms of specified sites. In this case, there is a further subdivision with subblocks for each site; so, for example, codes C15–C26 are the malignant neoplasms of the digestive organs.

Chapter XX covers external causes of morbidity and mortality. So, for example, W29 is the three-character code for *an injury due to contact with powered hand tools and domestic machinery* (including, rather frighteningly, spin-dryers). For many of the codes, but not, mercifully, W29, a further level of classification is provided in a fourth character.

The codes A80–A89 are assigned to the viral infections of the central nervous system, with A81 being the *slow viral infections of the central nervous system* and A81.0 being *Creutzfeldt–Jakob disease*. Most of the definitions are very succinct statements of inclusion and exclusion criteria but they can be quite lengthy. See *Asperger's syndrome* (a relatively new addition to the classification) in Box 7.1 for an example.

In certain circumstances a user may wish to describe a condition using two ICD-10 codes. The classification's designers anticipate two such kinds of situation. The first is where the user wishes to use a diagnostic code for an underlying disease in conjunction with a code for a manifestation of the disease in a particular site, where the manifestation is a problem in its own right. This is clearly linked to the practice in the issuing of death certificates where

Table 7.1 The division of ICD-10 codes into chapters.

Chapter	Codes	Description
I	A00-B99	Certain infectious and parasitic diseases
II	C00-D48	Neoplasms
III	D50-D89	Diseases of the blood, blood-forming organs and certain diseases of the immune system
IV	E00-E90	Endocrine, nutritional and metabolic disorders
V	F00-F99	Mental and behavioural disorders
VI	G00-G99	Diseases of the nervous system
VII	H00-H59	Diseases of the eye and adnexa
VIII	H60-H95	Diseases of the ear and mastoid process
IX	I00-I99	Diseases of the circulatory system
X	J00-J99	Diseases of the respiratory system
XI	K00-K93	Diseases of the digestive system
XII	L00-L99	Diseases of the skin and subcutaneous system
XIII	M00-M99	Diseases of the musculoskeletal system and connective tissue
XIV	N00-N99	Diseases of the genitourinary system
XV	O00-O99	Diseases of pregnancy, childbirth and puerperium
XVI	P00-P96	Certain conditions originating in the perinatal period
XVII	Q00-Q99	Congenital malformations, deformations and chromosomal abnormalities
XVIII	R00-R99	Symptoms, signs and abnormal clinical and laboratory findings not elsewhere classified
XIX	S00-T98	Injury, poisoning and certain other consequences of external causes
XX	V01-Y98	External causes of morbidity and mortality
XXI	Z00-Z99	Factors influencing health status and contact with services

immediate and underlying causes of death are both recorded. For example, G22 is the code for *Parkinsonism in diseases classified elsewhere* and A52.1 is the code for *symptomatic neurosyphilis*. The expectation behind the definition of G22 is clearly that it will be used in conjunction with codes such as A52.1. The second way in which users are invited to combine codes is where a second code is required to fully describe a condition; for example, the definition of *autism* includes a suggestion that a second code be used to indicate the degree of mental retardation.

There are a number of difficulties with ICD-10. The arrangement of concepts in a single hierarchy means that arbitrary choices have to be made about where certain concepts must go. If a cancer is to be listed in Chapter II under neoplasms, it cannot be listed under any of the anatomical locations covered in Chapters VI to XIV. Breast cancer is not, according to ICD-10, a disease of the breast.

The fact that the classification works by simply enumerating the concepts to be covered means that updating the classification is difficult. For example, if CJD is A81.0, then, if nvCJD is a new and distinct disease, we might rationally want it to appear at A81.1 in a future classification, but that code has already been used.

Box 7.1 The definition of Asperger's Syndrome given in ICD-10

F84.5 Asperger's Syndrome
A disorder of uncertain nosological validity, characterised by the same
kind of qualitative abnormalities of reciprocal social interaction that
typify autism, together with a restricted, stereotyped, repetitive
repertoire of interests and activities. The disorder differs from autism
primarily in that there is no general delay or retardation in language or
in cognitive development. Most individuals are of normal general
intelligence but it is common for them to be markedly clumsy; the
condition occurs predominately in boys (in a ratio of about eight boys to
one girl). It seems highly likely that at least some cases represent mild
varieties of autism, but it is uncertain whether or not that is so for all.
There is a strong tendency for the abnormalities to persist into
adolescence and adult life and it seems that they represent individual
characteristics that are not greatly affected by environmental influences.
Psychotic episodes occasionally occur in early adult life.

Diagnostic Guidelines
Diagnosis is based on the combination of a lack of any clinically
significant general delay in language or cognitive development plus, as
with autism, the presence of qualitative deficiencies in reciprocal social
interaction and restricted, repetitive, stereotyped patterns of behaviour,
interests and activities. There may or may not be problems in
communication similar to those associated with autism, but significant
language retardation would rule out the diagnosis.

Includes:
  • autistic psychopathy
  • schizoid disorder of childhood

Excludes:
  • anakastic personality disorder
  • attachment disorders of childhood
  • obsessive–compulsive disorder
  • schizotypical disorder
  • simple schizophrenia

In fact the issue of nvCJD is an interesting one. As things stand one could
put it with CJD in A81.0 but there is also code A81.8, defined as *other slow
infection of the central nervous system*, and one A81.9 defined as *slow infection of
the central nervous system not otherwise specified*. The existence of such categories
is troubling because their scope is determined by what is left over from other
concepts and therefore will change as other concepts are added or redefined.
They cannot be interpreted in isolation from the rest of the classification.

Box 7.2 The definition of disease

Homosexuality was removed from ICD-10 only in 1992. Its definition as an illness had been removed from the American Psychiatric Association's *Diagnostic and Statistical Manual of Mental Disorders* somewhat sooner, in 1974. That decision had, however, been controversial and many psychiatrists and psychologists continued in their attempts to cure patients of their homosexuality. The most common treatment was electric shock aversion therapy[1]. Electrodes were attached to the patient's wrist or lower leg. He (it generally was 'he', lesbians were rarely treated for their 'condition') then looked at photographs of men and women in various stages of undress. Patients would receive shocks when looking at pictures of men, and avoid shocks by moving to photographs of women. Smith *et al.*'s oral history of the treatment of homosexuality in Britain identified a patient who received this therapy as recently as 1980.

The debate about what is and what is not a disease is particularly charged in psychiatry because it deals with behaviour and social norms. Although homosexuality is no longer considered a disease, other sexual behaviours that are transgressive without being obviously harmful are still considered as diseases. For example, the MeSH terms class transvestism as a sexual dysfunction. To take a different area of behaviour, the section of the Read Codes that deals with disorders has a category for 'Harmful Substance Use' under which alcohol and cannabis are listed but not tobacco. Smoking does, however, figure in the Read Codes as a Health-Related Behaviour and as a Dependence Syndrome.

Difficult questions about what is and what is not disease occur throughout medicine. Women who develop a breast lump that turns out not to be cancer are sometimes said to have a form of 'benign breast disease'. However, it is not clear that all patients in this condition can appropriately be said to be suffering from a disease. The breast can develop symptoms similar to those of cancer through processes of normal change and equally through processes which although not 'normal' do not require treatment. High blood pressure is sometimes considered a disease, sometimes as a risk factor for forms of cardiovascular disease.

The concept of disease does seem to be linked to that of normality. If something is normal, then we do not think of it as a disease. The term 'normal', however, is a complex one. It has a specific meaning within statistics where it refers to a particular distribution of probabilities. The phrase 'normal range', which seems to be derived from this meaning, refers to the two standard deviations above and below the mean of a distribution; so for any measure, the bottom 2.5% and the top 2.5% of the population are outside the 'normal range'. Clearly, it does not follow that every time we devise a new way of measuring people, we must then classify 5% of the population as diseased. Outside of statistics, 'normal' is sometimes used to mean 'common' or 'representative'. On other occasions its meaning is different again; if we now say that homosexuality (or come to that left-handedness) is perfectly normal, we do not mean that it is not unusual, but something else: that it is harmless or perhaps that it is acceptable.

Murphy identifies a number of other ways in which one might attempt to define disease[2]. One thought might be that it is the response of the body to harmful or threatening insults. This, however, would exclude congenital disorders and include benign responses such as suntan. One could define disease as something that might shorten a patient's life or threaten their happiness, but again that would include things that are not really diseases (poverty, ignorance, recklessness).

There does not seem to be an easy answer. Murphy links the definition of disease to the concept of homeostasis. We are able to function in a range of environments and to survive a variety of stresses because our bodies incorporate mechanisms that respond to these external challenges. These regulatory mechanisms promote homeostasis, a return towards optimal operating conditions. Certainly it is true that many patients present in clinic because their bodies have proved unable to deal with some environmental challenge. Murphy argues that the term disease is used in three distinct senses, each to do with the interaction between the organism and its environment:

1 The body's attempt to maintain a normal operating environment despite external stresses. So the symptoms of food poisoning are, essentially, a homeostatic process. The appropriate treatment is to work with the homeostatic process.
2 Perversion of a normal homeostatic process. Hypertension is an example of this. The appropriate treatment is to adjust the homeostatic process.
3 An anarchical state that is no way directed towards serving the body. Cancer is the obvious example here. The treatment is to attack the anarchic system.

This does not entirely solve the problem. One grey area that remains concerns asymptomatic patients in whom a process is underway which may lead to disease. Are such patients suffering from an early stage of the disease or are they healthy but at risk? It does, however, help get away from a discussion of normality and normal behaviour or normal functioning. The important point about homeostasis is that it is defined in terms of what is optimal for the individual in dealing with their environment, not in terms of what is normal.

(continued)

> **Box 7.2 The definition of disease** (*continued*)
>
> ## References
>
> 1. Smith G, Bartlett A, King M. Treatments of homosexuality in Britain since the 1950s – an oral history: the experience of patients. *BMJ* 2004;328:427.
> 2. Murphy EA. *The Logic of Medicine*. Baltimore, MD: Johns Hopkins University Press, 1976.

ICD-10 makes a distinction between *not elsewhere specified* and *not elsewhere classified*. The form of words *not elsewhere specified* is intended to deal with a situation that often crops up in medical terminology, when there are different forms of a condition one of which is very much more common than the others. In these situations. it often happens that the name that rationally should be the umbrella term for all the conditions is loosely applied to the common one, so that the term *mitral stenosis* is assumed to refer to *rheumatic mitral stenosis*, unless it is further qualified; hence it figures in the classification as *mitral stenosis, not elsewhere specified*. The form of words *not elsewhere classified* is used as a warning, to indicate that there are other categories for this condition, elsewhere in the classification. For example, J16 is defined as *pneumonia due to other infectious organism not elsewhere classified*, because there are many other categories of pneumonia elsewhere, e.g. P23, *congenital pneumonia*.

MeSH: Medical Subject Headings

Since 1966 the National Library of Medicine in the USA has been compiling indexes of published medical research. The result, Medline, was described in Chapter 4. It is a fantastic resource for medical research, a database of 12 million citations covering 4600 medical journals published in 70 countries. There are a variety of ways of getting hold of Medline, but for most purposes the simplest is the Entrez PubMed website. Using PubMed you can search Medline in a variety of ways: if you are looking for a particular article and you know who wrote it, for example, you simply enter the authors' names, perhaps a range of dates, and, with luck, PubMed will retrieve the complete citation, an abstract and even, if you're really lucky, a link to an electronic version of the complete text of the article. When I use PubMed, it is generally not to find a specific article that I am already aware of, but just to find what articles have been published on a particular topic. One can do this in a slightly hit-or-miss way by just entering a few likely words in the search box – just as one would with Google or any of the other Internet search engines – and seeing what comes up. The alternative is to take more careful note of the work that the National Institutes of Health (NIH) put into indexing Medline and to search using the Medical Subject Headings (MeSH).

Table 7.2 The top-level headings in the MeSH hierarchy.

A	Anatomy
B	Organisms
C	Diseases
D	Chemicals and drugs
E	Analytical, diagnostic and therapeutic techniques and equipment
F	Psychiatry and psychology
G	Biological sciences
H	Physical sciences
I	Anthropology, education, sociology and social phenomena
J	Technology and food and beverages
K	Humanities
L	Information science
M	Persons
N	Health care
O	Geographic locations

Every year more than 400 000 articles are added to the database. When an article is added, it is indexed under a set of headings. This means that someone, an actual human being, has read it, decided what the article is about and how best to classify this 'aboutness' under a set of standard headings. These headings are the MeSH terms[2]

Multiple hierarchies

The MeSH terms cover a wider terrain than the ICD-10 codes, since the requirement here is to provide a set of categories that allows the classification of all biomedical research, whereas the authors of ICD-10 are essentially interested in causes of death and forms of illness. Table 7.2 shows the top-level headings in the MeSH hierarchy, and gives a sense of the scope of the classification.

The MeSH descriptors are, like the ICD-10 codes, arranged in a hierarchy. Each point in the hierarchy has a 'tree number'. When you go down a level in the hierarchy, each new descriptor has a tree number that consists of the tree number for the higher level with an additional suffix. So, for example, the tree number for Mental Disorders is F03, and one of the subclasses of Mental Disorders is Delirium, Dementia, Amnestic and Cognitive Disorders, which has the tree number F03.087. Dementia has the tree number F03.087.400; AIDS Dementia Complex is F03.087.400.050; and so on.

The MeSH hierarchy is more complicated than that of ICD-10. Whereas each ICD-10 code corresponds to a unique position in the hierarchy, a single MeSH term may occur in a number of places. A straightforward treelike decomposition of medical concepts is harder to make work in practice than it might seem at first glance. This is because there are many different ways in which concepts like diseases can be organised in a hierarchy. To go back to AIDS Dementia Complex, this concept appears not only under Mental Disorders [F03] but also under Diseases [C]. In fact it appears in four different places in

Table 7.3 AIDS Dementia Complex appears at five different locations in the hierarchy.

Virus Diseases [C02]
  RNA Virus Infections [C02.782]
    Retroviridae Infections [C02.782.815]
      Lentivirus Infections [C02.782.815.616]
        HIV Infections [C02.782.815.616.400]
                          AIDS Dementia Complex [C02.782.815.616.400.070]
Virus Diseases [C02]
  Sexually Transmitted Diseases [C02.800]
    Sexually Transmitted Diseases, Viral [C02.800.801]
      HIV Infections [C02.800.801.400]
                          AIDS Dementia Complex [C02.800.801.400.070]
Nervous System Diseases [C10]
  Central Nervous System Diseases [C10.228]
    Brain Diseases [C10.228.140]
      Dementia [C10.228.140.380]
                          AIDS Dementia Complex [C10.228.140.380.070]
Immunologic Diseases [C20]
  Immunologic Deficiency Syndromes [C20.673]
    HIV Infections [C20.673.480]
                          AIDS Dementia Complex [C20.673.480.070]
Mental Disorders [F03]
  Delirium, Dementia, Amnestic, Cognitive Disorders [F03.087]
    Dementia [F03.087.400]
                          AIDS Dementia Complex [F03.087.400.050]

---

the Diseases hierarchy: once under Nervous System Diseases, once under Immunological Diseases and twice under Virus Diseases – once as an RNA Virus Infection and once as a Sexually Transmitted Disease. As is shown in Table 7.3, each appearance of the heading in the hierarchy has a different tree number. There is a separate code that uniquely identifies the heading, but the tree numbers correspond not to headings but to each appearance of a heading in the hierarchy. Here is another example to show how tangled the hierarchy is: fathers figure under [F] as a behaviour, under [I] as a topic for sociological enquiry and under [M] as a class of persons.

A further difference between ICD-10 and MeSH is that the MeSH hierarchy extends to an arbitrary number of levels. The ICD-10 hierarchy is relatively flat. Blocks of three-character codes are assigned to the 21 different chapters. There is little by way of structure within the chapters and for each three-character code there is a single layer of further specification provided by the fourth character. In contrast the tree of MeSH is allowed to extend to as many different levels of specialisation as the domain demands.

MeSH tables

Each heading is defined by a table. See Table 7.4, for example, which gives the heading, a list of tree numbers that identify the different points where the

Table 7.4 The complete MeSH entry for AIDS Dementia Complex.

MeSH heading	AIDS Dementia Complex
Tree number	C02.782.815.616.400.070
Tree number	C02.800.801.400.070
Tree number	C10.228.140.380.070
Tree number	C20.673.480.070
Tree number	F03.087.400.050
Annotation	Coord IM with HIV-1 or HIV-2 (IM or NIM) if pertinent
Scope note	A neurologic condition associated with the Acquired Immuno-deficiency Syndrome and characterised by impaired concentration and memory, slowness of hand movements, ataxia, incontinence, apathy and gait difficulties associated with HIV-1 viral infection of the central nervous system. Pathologic examination of the brain reveals white matter rarefication, perivascular infiltrates of lymphocytes, foamy macrophages and multinucleated giant cells. (From Adams *et al. Principles of Neurology*, 6th edn, pp. 760–761; *N Engl J Med* 1995;332(14):934–940.)
Entry term	AIDS Encephalopathy
Entry term	Dementia Complex, AIDS-Related
Entry term	HIV Dementia
Entry term	HIV Encephalopathy
Entry term	HIV-1-Associated Cognitive Motor Complex
Entry term	HIV-Associated Cognitive Motor Complex
Entry term	AIDS-Related Dementia Complex
Entry term	Acquired Immunodeficiency Syndrome Dementia Complex
Entry term	Dementia Complex, Acquired Immunodeficiency Syndrome
Entry term	Encephalopathy, AIDS
Entry term	Encephalopathy, HIV
Entry term	HIV-1 Cognitive and Motor Complex
Allowable qualifiers	BL CF CI CL CO DH DI DT EC EH EM EN EP ET GE HI IM ME MI MO NU PA PC PP PS PX RA RH RI RT SU TH TM UR US VE VI
Previous indexing	Acquired Immunodeficiency Syndrome (1983–1989)
Previous indexing	Dementia (1983–1989)
History note	1990
Unique ID	D015526

heading appears in the hierarchy, some information about annotation, a brief note explaining the scope of the term, a set of what are called entry terms, a set of what are called qualifiers, some information about how the heading was indexed in earlier versions of the system and a unique ID. The next two subsections discuss the idea of entry terms and the system of qualifiers.

Multiple entry points

Each heading corresponds to what the MeSH developers call a descriptor class. A descriptor class might be a single concept, but it might correspond to a cluster of concepts. So, for example, the descriptor AIDS Dementia Complex refers to that concept, but also to a refinement of it, HIV encephalopathy, and also to a

Table 7.5 The various entry points for AIDS Dementia Complex.

AIDS DEMENTIA COMPLEX [descriptor class]
Concept Class I – preferred concept
Terms:
AIDS Dementia Complex (preferred term)
HIV Dementia
HIV-Associated Cognitive Motor Complex
Dementia Complex, AIDS-Related
Concept Class II – Subordinate Concept (narrower)
Terms:
HIV Encephalopathy (preferred term)
AIDS Encephalopathy
Concept Class III – Subordinate Concept (related)
Terms:
HIV-1-Associated Cognitive Motor Complex (preferred term)

related concept, HIV-1-Associated Cognitive Motor Complex. Some of these concepts are associated with more than one term. For example, HIV Encephalopathy can be referred to either using the preferred term (which, unsurprisingly, is HIV Encephalopathy) or a synonym: AIDS Encephalopathy. The complete list of terms for the concept and for all the subordinate and related concepts provides the total set of possible entry points for the heading Aids Dementia Complex (Table 7.5). That is to say, searching PubMed for AIDS Encephalopathy will retrieve all the articles indexed under AIDS Dementia Complex.

Qualifiers

As well as being associated with a set of alternative entry points, each heading is associated with a list of allowable qualifiers. These let the reader who indexed the article specify the theme of each article more precisely. So, to pick an article at random from the 2245 articles indexed under AIDS Dementia Complex:

> Nath A, Maragos WF, Avison MJ, Schmitt FA, Berger JR. Acceleration of HIV dementia with methamphetamine and cocaine. *J Neurovirol* 2001;7(1):66–71.

is indexed under the following headings, with the indicated qualifiers shown after slashes (asterisk indicates heading is a major subject for the article):

MH – AIDS Dementia Complex/complications/*diagnosis
MH – Adult
MH – Amphetamine-Related Disorders/complications/*diagnosis
MH – Antiretroviral Therapy, Highly Active
MH – Blood–Brain Barrier
MH – Brain/pathology
MH – Case Report

MH – Cholinergic Antagonists/therapeutic use
MH – Cocaine-Related Disorders/complications/*diagnosis
MH – Disease Progression
MH – Human
MH – Levodopa/therapeutic use
MH – Magnetic Resonance Imaging
MH – Male
MH – Methamphetamine/adverse effects
MH – Movement Disorders/complications/diagnosis/drug therapy
MH – Support, US Government, Public Health Service

The system of qualifiers allows users who wish to search for articles about, for example, the adverse effects of methamphetamine to avoid retrieving articles about its therapeutic uses.

Read Codes

The best-known coding system, at least in the UK, is that of Read Codes. It was first developed by James Read in the 1980s, for use in general practice. In the first version each term was associated with a four-character code. Although the labels were not meaningful abbreviations, they carried information about the position of the term in the hierarchy. So all examinations and signs began with a 2, all observations relating to fever began with 2E, all those relating to the level of fever began with 2E3 and the code for 'elevated temperature' was 2E34.

Just as the UK ran out of seven-digit telephone numbers in the 1990s, so James Read had to move to a five-character code in order to expand his system for hospital use. This five-byte set was later updated to create Version 2. Version 3, also known as Clinical Terms Version 3 (The Read Codes) – or CTV3 for short – followed in 1994[3]. The next version, SNOMED CT, is an amalgamation of the Read Codes with the US SNOMED system and is the final system discussed in this chapter.

Despite the enormous investment that was put into the development of the Read Codes (see Box 7.3) they are hardly used outside primary care and are used only in fairly limited ways within primary care. Interestingly, the most well-developed version of the Read Codes, CTV3, is hardly used at all, with most commercial developers of GP software choosing not to upgrade beyond Version 2. This is disappointing because research has shown clear advantages to using CTV3[4]. These advantages were, however, not obvious enough, or not well understood or too removed from actual patient benefit to push forward the adoption of a new system. The clinicians did not demand it, the developers were not keen to provide it and the government did not force the issue, and then SNOMED CT appeared on the horizon, so the move to CTV3 never really happened.

CTV3 is, however, still worthy of our attention because it is worth looking in detail at three innovations that were introduced in moving to CTV3: the

Box 7.3 The purchase of the Read Codes

Maria Eagle MP: *Mr Langlands, if you saw someone walk into a brick wall, pick themselves up and walk into that same brick wall again, and pick themselves up and walk into the brick wall again, would the thought maybe cross your mind that they might be drunk or of unsound mind or would you perhaps conclude that they were incapable of avoiding brick walls?*

Alan Langlands: *I think I know the next question and therefore I fashion my answer accordingly. I think that this Committee has heard on a number of occasions about failings in relation to information management and technology in the NHS Executive and in the NHS.*

Minutes of Evidence to the House of Commons Public Accounts Committee, 23 March 1998:

The Read Codes were originally developed by the eponymous Dr Read. However, in 1990 the copyright was acquired by the NHS. The further development of the Codes was paid for by the NHS, which established the NHS Centre for Coding and Classification (the Centre) for that purpose. Distribution of, and support for, the Codes was, however, the responsibility of a private company, to whom users of the codes had to pay a licence fee. The curious feature of the arrangement was that Dr Read was both the director of the Centre and the owner of the company, Computer-Aided Medical Systems (CAMS), granted exclusive rights to distribute the Codes.

By the time the project came to the attention of the Public Accounts Committee, Dr Read, who had already received £1.25 million for the original sale of the Read Codes, was being paid over £70,000 a year as director of the Centre at which £32 million of public money had been spent developing the Codes, the use of which was earning him at least £40,000 a year through his company. There were some juicy details in the evidence to the committee, with questions being asked about the appointment of Dr Read's brother – a primary school teacher – to a £40,000 post in CAMS and about the promotion of a member of the Centre's staff with whom Dr Read had a personal relationship. At one point, it was noted, Dr Read's travel expenses were being paid twice over: once through the Centre and once through CAMS.

Unsurprisingly the Committee's Report concluded that the NHS Executive had failed to exercise effective oversight in financial and management matters at the Centre and had set in place arrangements that created a conflict of interest for Dr Read. Their report also highlighted a number of findings that the committee felt were of general applicability and that are directly relevant to the subject of this book:

- The need to plan investment in information technology on the basis of sound investment appraisals. The report argued that the NHS Executive failed to assess the cost and benefits, to analyse the risks or to produce a business case for the project on which it went on to spend £32 million.
- The need to evaluate pilot projects before implementation. The NHS Executive was said to have been reluctant to agree to a full independent appraisal of the Read Codes before implementation.

The tragedy in all this was that the same committee had made not dissimilar points about previous projects, most notoriously the Wessex Regional Health Authority Regional Information Systems Plan. This was a project that aimed to install terminals in all offices, hospitals and wards in the Wessex region. All core systems, covering hospital information, manpower, estates, community care and accountancy, were to be accessible from any terminal, and data in any application would be accesible by any other. Implementation was expected to take five years at a cost of £25.8 million. When the project was finally abandoned, in 1990, £20 million had been wasted, little had been implemented: a ledger system, accounts systems in five districts, and a hospital information system in one single hospital.

In concluding its report into the purchase of the Read Codes, the Committee wrote: 'Clear lessons have emerged from the development of the Read Codes, about setting out business cases about project and programme management and about implementation of systems across the NHS. We look to the Executive to apply these lessons to other areas of their Information Management and Technology Strategy.' It would be interesting to know if those responsible felt that these lessons had been applied in more recent projects.

Reference

1. Public Accounts Committee. *Public Accounts Sixty-Second Report*. London: House of Commons, 1998.

distinction between concepts and terms; the use of multiple hierarchies; and the idea of qualifiers. These innovations are of technical interest and are also of practical relevance because they are retained in SNOMED CT.

Concepts, descriptions and terms

CTV3 makes a distinction between the concepts used in medicine and the terms that are used to describe them. We say that the terms *tumour* and *neoplasm* are synonyms because they are used to describe the same concept. Just as two or more terms can apply to a single concept, sometimes two

Table 7.6 Read Codes and Term IDs. The two concepts of umbilical and spinal cord compression are both described by two terms: a preferred term and a synonym. The term *Cord compression* applies to two concepts.

Read Code	Term	P/S	Term ID
X40Cc	Umbilical cord compression	P	YaaGm
X40Cc	Cord compression	S	Y40xj
Xa0Nk	Spinal cord compression	P	Ya1XS
Xa0Nk	Cord compression	S	Y40xj

concepts can be described by a single term. For example, the term *fit* can be used to describe convulsions but also a general state of well-being.

In CTV3 each concept is given a unique five-character code, the Read Code. Each term is also given a unique five-character code, the term ID. A descriptions file identifies which terms apply to each concept. As in the MeSH, where two or more terms describe a concept, one of the terms is identified as the preferred term (P) and the others are designated as synonyms (S) (Table 7.6).

Multiple hierarchies

The early versions of the Read Codes were, like ICD-10, essentially enumerative systems, where each concept was assigned a single code and the code was determined by the position that the concept was assigned in the hierarchy. In CTV3, however, as in MeSH, each concept may appear at more than one location in the hierarchy (Table 7.7). The code, therefore, is assigned to the concept, not to the position in the hierarchy. The concepts are assigned codes

Table 7.7 CTV3 includes multiple hierarchies, allowing a 'child' to have several 'parents'. For example, *tuberculous meningitis* is classified under *bacterial diseases* but also under *neurological disorders*.

Two fragments of the CTV3 concepts hierarchy
Disorders
Neurological disorders
Inflammatory and infective disorders of the CNS
Meningitis
Infective meningitis
Bacterial meningitis
Tuberculous meningitis
Infective disorder
Bacterial disease
Mycobacterial disease
Tuberculosis
Tuberculosis of meninges and CNS
Tuberculous meningitis

arbitrarily and then grouped into hierarchies that reflect the designers' model of the domain.

Qualifiers

In the clinical terms, as in other systems, concepts are organised hierarchically so that the concepts at the bottom of the hierarchy are more closely specified than those at the top. Each downward step through the hierarchy is a move from a more general to a more specific classification, perhaps corresponding to the addition of an adjective to the description of the disease or symptom or procedure. There are certain adjectives that are used to describe almost all disorders or almost all procedures. Almost all disorders, for example, have a severity (mild, moderate or severe). Almost all procedures have a priority (urgent or non-urgent). It makes sense, therefore, to treat these terms as adjectives, as terms that can be used to *qualify* concepts in the hierarchy. This is slightly different from the way qualifiers are used in MeSH. Here the qualifiers provide a further level of refinement; there the qualifiers provide a different set of axes for refinement.

The technique used in CTV3 is to allow users to construct triples composed of an object (the core concept), an attribute and a value. So, for example, a disorder such as migraine can have attributes: severity, episodicity and site. Severity can take the values mild, moderate and severe. Episodicity can take the values first episode, new episode, ongoing episode. Site can take any number of values identifying brain tissue structures. Each of the attributes and each of the values is itself a concept in the CTV3 hierarchy.

CTV3 contains a template for each concept. The template defines the set of legal combinations of attributes and values that are appropriate for the concept. For example, migraine may have the attribute site, but depression, for example, may not. Depression may take the attribute severity, while cancer may not. Interestingly breast cancer can take the attribute site, but cancer cannot. Remember that one of the goals of coding was to remove synonyms; therefore, systems like CTV3 are designed so that there is only one way to represent a concept. Since breast cancer is a core concept in the hierarchy, it must not be possible to create a qualified concept, *cancer: site = breast*.

SNOMED CT

The Systematized Nomenclature of Medicine (SNOMED) began life as the Systematized Nomenclature of Pathology (SNOP) and was an initiative of the American College of Pathologists begun in 1965. SNOP evolved into SNOMED in 1974 and went through four different versions before it was decided, in 1999, that the next version would be a merger between the existing SNOMED terminology and CTV3[5,6].

The basic unit in SNOMED CT, as in CTV3, is the concept. SNOMED CT contains more than 350 000 concepts. Each concept is given a unique identifier and a set of descriptions. The description is a word or form of words used in clinical language to denote the concept. Just as in the MeSH and the Read Codes, where there is more than one description for a concept, one is always considered the preferred term and the others are labelled as synonyms. There is a slight complication in SNOMED CT in that, in addition to the preferred term and the synonyms, each concept is also given a 'fully specified name'; generally this is an idealised version of the preferred term, which is slightly too long-winded to be acceptable in practice. For example, the descriptions provided for the concept identified as 22298006 are:

Fully specified name: Myocardial Infarction (disorder)
Preferred term: Myocardial Infarction
Synonym: Cardiac infarction
Synonym: Heart attack
Synonym: Infarction of heart
Synonym: Infarto de miocardio

Definitions

This may not seem too different from CTV3. SNOMED CT is, however, a very different system from CTV3. Unlike CTV3 or its predecessors, the terminology sets out to provide a set of definitions for each of the concepts in the domain. By 'definition' I mean something very far from 'description'. In SNOMED parlance the description is just a selection of text strings corresponding to possible synonyms. The definition is also something quite different from the paragraphs of explanatory text that accompany the more contentious terms in ICD-10. The SNOMED definition of a concept is part of the logic of the system; it is represented as the set of relationships that exist between the concept and the other concepts in the system.

There are two kinds of relationship in SNOMED: 'is a' links and 'attribute' links. The definition of a concept therefore has two parts: a set of 'is a' links between the concept and its parents and a set of 'attribute' links that connect it to other concepts. The 'is a' links specify the concept's position in one or more hierarchies. Already in MeSH and in CTV3 we have encountered the idea that a concept can be classified in different ways and therefore might be found in more than one position in a classification. This idea is taken further in SNOMED CT. Concepts are arranged in 19 hierarchies, listed in Table 7.8, and, of course, each concept is allowed to exist in more than one. So, for example, *lumbar discitis* is a *discitis* and also a *disorder of back*.

Attributes

The definition of a concept also includes a set of attributes: relationships that link the concept to other concepts in other hierarchies (Figure 7.2). For example, the definition of *lumbar discitis* includes the relationship Finding–Site, which connects the concept *lumbar discitis* to the concept *intervertebral*

Table 7.8 There are 3 major and 16 minor hierarchies in the SNOMED clinical terms.

SNOMED CT's 19 hierarchies	
Major	Finding
	Disease
	Procedure/intervention
Minor	Observable entity
	Body structure
	Organism
	Substance
	Pharmaceutical/biologic product
	Specimen
	Physical object
	Physical force
	Events
	Environments/geographical locations
	Social contexts
	Context-dependent categories
	Staging and scales
	Attribute
	Qualifier
	Special concept

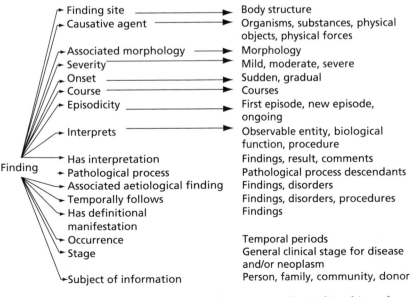

Figure 7.2 Attributes used in the definition of concepts in the Findings hierarchy.

disc. This connection is part of the definition of *lumbar discitis,* it is part of what gives the concept its meaning. The concept *allergic rhinitis due to pollen* contains the following definition:

Allergic rhinitis due to pollen

Is a	allergic rhinitis
Has finding site	nose
Has associated morphology	inflammation
Has causative agent	pollen

The definition consists of a single 'is a' link that identifies the concept, which is an immediate generalisation of *allergic rhinitis due to pollen* and of three attribute links that identify its essential characteristics.

It is worth reflecting on the intellectual journey involved in moving from a simple enumerative coding scheme like ICD-10 or the early versions of the Read Codes to a scheme like this. Instead of the terminology being a list of labelled concepts in which the only structure is the grouping together of concepts into chapters or sections that address a common theme, SNOMED CT employs a highly multidimensional representation in which different ways of classifying concepts in the domain are teased apart, allowing the explicit representation of concept definitions in terms of the relationships between concepts. To return to the molecular model metaphor introduced at the start of the chapter, SNOMED CT is not just an enumeration of the semantic 'atoms' but in fact a specification of how they are combined in 'molecules'. We do not just say that *lumbar discitis* is a term within the terminology, we have a scheme that says things about it: for example, that it occurs in the intervertebral disc.

The development of such a system is no mean feat. Identifying the appropriate links for the huge variety of concepts required by SNOMED is a task of enormous complexity and some subtlety. For example, the concept *repair of hammer toe* refers to a procedure for which in 90% of cases the most obvious parent is *incision of bone;* however, 90% still leaves the 10% of cases where the repair only involves soft tissue, hence the parent concept has to be the more general *surgical repair.* Similar niceties are involved in the assignment of relationships; the rule is that the relationship must hold true in 98% of cases. Clearly the modellers will not always have the data to hand that would allow them to know for certain whether it holds in 90%, 95% or 98% of cases. Clearly, too, things can change. There is another subtlety that makes the assignment of links even more complicated: the relationships that are assigned for a parent concept are automatically also held to be true of its children.

Qualifiers
SNOMED CT provides a similar mechanism to that provided by the qualifiers in CTV3 for allowing users to add further detail to the concepts provided in the standard. They can do this in two ways: they can add an attribute that was not previously included in the definition or they can edit an attribute so

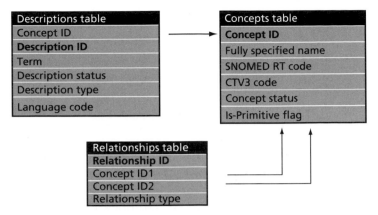

Figure 7.3 SNOMED CT database tables.

that it links the concept to a more specific class. An example of additional characterisation would be to add the attribute *priority* with value *emergency* to the list of attributes defining *appendectomy*. An example of further specification would be to change the definition of *bacterial meningitis* so that the causative agent was *streptococcus* rather than *bacterium*.

Although SNOMED CT is a much more sophisticated system for representing medical concepts than most of its predecessors, the design is relatively simple. The standard can be considered a set of just three database tables: Concepts, Descriptions and Relationships (Figure 7.3). Consider each in turn, starting with the table of Concepts. Each concept has a unique identifier. Each identifier has a row in the Concepts table containing the corresponding identifiers from the two legacy systems SNOMED RT and CTV3, the concept status (active or retired) and a flag indicating if the concept is currently considered to be fully defined. Each identifier also has a row in the Descriptions table, which includes all the descriptions that correspond to the concept. The Descriptions table has a row for each concept, and a column for the fully specified name, a column for the preferred name and as many extra columns as are required, one for each of the synonyms. Finally the Relationships table will have four columns: a relationship ID, the concept IDs for the two concepts in the relationship and a relationship type. Essentially, the type tells us whether the relationship is an 'is a' link, i.e. part of the hierarchical arrangement of concepts, or an 'attribute', a connection across two hierarchies.

Desiderata for a controlled clinical terminology

In 1998, James Cimino set out a number of desiderata for a controlled clinical terminology[7]. The single most important quality of any terminology is, obviously, coverage. Nothing is more important than that there should be a code in the terminology to express what the user wishes to record. Of course, there are different ways of achieving adequate coverage. The straightforward enumeration of concepts is probably not adequate; some degree of compositionality is required, either combining atomic codes or allowing modifiers to add a further level of specification. In addition to coverage, Cimino identifies a number of desiderata connected to the role of concepts in terminologies: first, that we should understand that the unit of symbolic processing is the concept; second, that the concepts should be permanent and inviolate even if the hierarchy or the descriptive terms used are required to change; and finally, that each concept should have a unique identifier, which is one of the descriptive terms for the concept, not, as it is in ICD-10 and was in the Read Codes until CTV3, a number derived from the concept's position in the hierarchy. Hierarchies are almost universal in the field of clinical terminology and most systems, MeSH, CTV3 and SNOMED included, adopt multiple hierarchies which allow a child to have many parents. As was noted in the discussion of ICD-10, concepts such as Not Elsewhere Classified are problematic and a particular barrier to the graceful evolution of the terminology, and any system with ambitions to survive even a short period should be designed to allow for changes and revisions. A further desideratum is that the terminology should support a variety of levels of granularity, coping with the varying degrees of precision required by different authors. A related idea is that the terminology should support a variety of views, with different users being shown more or less of the building blocks that make up the terminology. The implication here is that there will be parts in the hierarchy that might normally be concealed from view. There might be 'intermediate' concepts that are required to allow a sensible decomposition from top-level concepts to meaningful specific concepts but that are not, in practice, useful descriptors for clinical concepts. There is a set of requirements for a terminology that is to do with how much of the internal machinery is exposed to the user. By machinery, I mean not just the 'intermediate concepts' mentioned above but other elements too, such as the formal concept definitions of the kind provided in SNOMED CT.

Most of these desiderata have been met by the later systems, CTV3 and SNOMED CT. It is interesting, however, that the older systems are still widely used and there seems very little sign that manufacturers wish to adopt the newer proposals or that their customers are putting them under any pressure to move on. The advantages of the newer systems are in part technical; they are more elegant solutions. This is, however, irrelevant if people have adapted to the inadequacies of the earlier systems. They are also more powerful tools. They are more expressive, allowing users to put more clinical content into codes. They also have a richer internal structure, allowing closer integration with other tools, such as decision support systems. These advantages, however, remain largely theoretical. Clinicians are not keen to put more effort into coding. Decision support tools to take advantage of the newer codes do not yet exist.

Chapter 8 looks at issues of knowledge representation, of how to represent concepts and ideas in computer systems. The techniques covered include those required to build the decision support tools, which are expected to allow coded patient data to be used to improve patient care. It is worth noting that these techniques are also used in the more sophisticated terminology systems, such as SNOMED CT. Interestingly, one of the more highly developed schemes for representing clinical knowledge (GALEN) is intended as a terminology server, a system that provides a set of rules and a representation of clinical concepts in order to be able to generate different terminologies for different clinical goals. To understand how this works, however, we will need to spend a little time looking at the notion of knowledge representation more generally.

References

1. World Health Organization. *International Statistical Classification of Diseases and Related Health Problems*, 1989 Revision. Geneva: World Health Organization, 1992.
2. National Library of Medicine. *Medical Subject Headings*. http://www.nlm.nih.gov/mesh/meshhome.html (accessed on 12 February 2004).
3. NHS Information Authority. *The Clinical Terms Version 3 (The Read Codes)*. Crown Copyright 2000.
4. Brown PJ, Warmington V, Laurence M, Prevost AT. Randomised crossover trial comparing the performance of Clinical Terms Version 3 and Read Codes 5 byte set coding schemes in general practice. *BMJ* 2003;326(7399):1127.
5. Snomed International. *Welcome To SNOMED*. http://www.snomed.org (accessed on 12 February 2004).
6. Snomed International. *SNOMED Clinical Terms User Guide*. American College of Pathologists, 2003.
7. Cimino JJ. Desiderata for controlled medical vocabularies in the twenty-first century. *Methods Inf Med* 1998;37:394–403.

CHAPTER 8
Knowledge representation

The term 'knowledge representation' comes from artificial intelligence, the attempt to program computers to carry out various tasks that, at least when carried out by humans, seem to require intelligence. Such tasks very often involve reasoning about a body of knowledge, perhaps very general knowledge about some aspect of the world, human behaviour or language, or some very specific knowledge about a particular domain. Inevitably, tackling such tasks with computers requires that the knowledge be rendered explicit in a computable formalism. The field of knowledge representation developed out of attempts to design such formalisms. Now, however, ideas that were first used in artificial intelligence are applied in other areas of computer science and knowledge representation is a field of more general interest.

One textbook on the topic defines knowledge representation as the application of logic and ontology to the task of constructing computable models for some domain[1]. We first met the term ontology in Chapter 2 where I said it was 'borrowed from a branch of philosophy concerned with questions of what kinds of thing can be said to exist'. In knowledge representation we are concerned with how we organise the often vague and unanalysed ideas that people have into a computable model of an application domain. Part of that process, the ontology part, is to do with working out what symbols and terms we need in the representation. The issues here are similar to those that were discussed in Chapter 7. The other part, the logic part, is to do with ensuring that the model is computable. The aim in this chapter is to focus more on the logic and less on the ontology, although a complete separation of the issues is impossible.

In introducing the term ontology in Chapter 2, I went on to say that 'in health informatics (and computer science more generally) the word is used to refer to a specification of the concepts and relationships that can exist for a particular domain and application'. In this chapter, I illustrate some of the important issues in knowledge representation by looking at examples of ontologies created for different clinical applications. First, I want to describe an initiative known as the Semantic Web, because the project provides a useful illustration of the challenges involved in building systems based on the representation of some body of knowledge and because some of the tools developed for the Semantic Web are becoming widely used in building ontologies for medicine and other fields.

Developing the Web

One of the enduring peculiarities of the information technology industry is that many of its most successful products provide solutions to problems that people did not know they had. No one knew that they needed a spreadsheet until Bricklin and Frankston invented Visicalc in the 1970s. No one knew that they really wanted email until DARPANET came along. The creation, by Tim Berners-Lee, of a system to allow the retrieval of structured documents stored on networked computers brought into being a medium that is now so ubiquitous that it takes an effort of mind to recall how unanticipated was its success[2]. The protocols and conventions that define the World Wide Web – that everything is identified via a uniform resource locator (URL), that the layout of documents is determined by a set of tags known as hypertext mark-up language (HTML), that files are transferred according to the hypertext transfer protocol (HTTP) – were designed by Berners-Lee in 1990 while he was working at the Conseil Européen pour la Recherche Nucléaire (CERN), the European organisation for nuclear research. The original objective was merely to develop document management facilities to help the institute's scientists. The first graphical user interface for a Web browser was developed by a graduate student at the United States National Center for Supercomputing Applications 3 years later. Netscape Communications was founded in April 1994, released its first browser – Netscape Navigator 1.0 – in December that year and was floated on Wall Street in August 1995, at which point it was valued at $2.7 billion.

Tim Berners-Lee subsequently moved to the Massachusetts Institute of Technology (MIT) and worked with a group known as the World Wide Web Consortium or W3C. The avowed aim of W3C is to allow the Web to achieve its full potential, and it works with a great many collaborators across the world developing new languages and standards to enhance the Web's capabilities. It is involved in a great many activities, and it would not be appropriate to list them all here. Broadly speaking, however, one can identify two ways in which the Web can be developed. I tend to think of HTML and HTTP as operating at a particular conceptual level, providing a layer above that of the nuts-and-bolts hardware and software that allow the retrieval and display of Web pages, and below that of the business and social processes that operate via the Web, such as booking plane tickets, browsing news headlines and downloading MP3s. One of the ways in which W3C seeks to develop the Web is to work down from that layer, extending the standards and protocols that define the Web so that they provide more control over the operation of the machines on which the software runs. This kind of work is aimed at making it possible for software applications to operate across the Web, providing what are known as Web services. Another way of enhancing the Web's capabilities is to extend the Web layer in the other direction, away from the detail required to program the computer and to look more at the concerns and goals of the human users. Traditional HTML tags serve to indicate how a document is laid out. Imagine if, instead of HTML, we used a mark-up language where the tags indicated what the document meant. Today's Web browsers parse the HTML tags that make up a Web page in order to be able to present it for human consumption. Imagine if, instead, the software we used to search the Web was able to process the information inherent in the tagged data and ascertain enough of the meaning to decide on its value or relevance. This is the goal of the Semantic Web[3].

The Semantic Web

Consider an example of how the Semantic Web might work. A medical researcher wishing to publish the protocol for a new clinical trial could choose to put it on the Web. Today he or she could do this by using HTML tags to define how a Web page could be laid out to make it accessible to a human reader. The tags define, for example, which bits of text should be displayed in bold or in italics, when paragraph breaks should be inserted, the use of tables and so on. With Semantic Web technology the researcher could choose to create a data file using tags that indicated which data items identified the researchers, the inclusion criteria, the aims of the study, the baseline tests to be performed, the details of the treatments to be compared and so on. Such a data file could not only be read by a human being but could also be analysed by some appropriate software tool. One of the big problems in medical research at the moment is maximising recruitment to clinical trials. Patients are often keen to participate in trials, and in theory clinicians want to see patients recruited into trials but nevertheless the opportunity is often missed. A number of large databases of clinical trials exist and are accessible via the Web. Imagine, however, if those databases were available via the Semantic Web. Instead of searching using a traditional search engine, a clinician with a patient who was just starting a new treatment could use a tool that was able to identify the tags used to describe clinical trials. The tool would be able to inspect the contents of clinical trials websites and automatically identify those that were most appropriate for a given patient.

Several things have to be put in place before this can be made to work. The most important, perhaps, is that the clinician, or rather his or her search engine, needs to have some way of identifying the medical researcher as someone whose website provides trusted content. Trust and proof are key concepts in the Semantic Web. At a more prosaic level, the search engine needs to be able to recognise the tags used to identify the different data items that make up the trial protocol. How can this work? How can we arrange it so that the software used by the clinician can anticipate how the medical re-searcher will have structured the data? One way would be for a body such as the W3C to decide on an appropriate set of tags and decree that everyone should use them, that they form a standard. The problem is that the tags would have to be very specific, to do with the detail of clinical trials, and the Semantic Web is intended to allow the representation of all sorts of data, from football scores to supermarket prices to the location of petrol stations.

The Semantic Web, therefore, has to operate in a highly decentralised way, just like the rest of the Web. To make this possible, the standards must be at a higher level than that of the domain-specific tags.

The first standard that needs to be defined is a mechanism for creating new kinds of tag. This is already in place. The extensible mark-up language (XML) is an easily understood and widely used formalism that allows users to mark up data files by creating their own tags. These tags define what the data are; in our example they specify that the various entries in the data file identify the relevant features of a clinical trial. The tags provide data about data and are therefore known as metadata. XML provides a syntax for creating metadata. The technologies that are being developed for the Semantic Web are in essence techniques that allow groups of users to work together by sharing metadata. To make the Semantic Web work we also need a standard way of using XML to make simple statements about a domain; for example, that this document is a clinical trial protocol, that Dr X is the author of this document etc. For the Semantic Web this is provided by the Resource Description Framework (RDF), a set of rules for providing simple descriptive information. In RDF, a notation based on triples – expressed in XML – allows you to assert that an object has a property with a value. So, for example, we might want to say that a document 'Clinical Trial of New Medication for Digital Ulcers Caused by Scleroderma' has a property 'created on', which might take the value '10 February 2004'. In RDF parlance, the document is the *object*, the property is a *predicate* and the value is the *subject*. Each element of the triple must be given a unique resource identifier (URI, a similar notion to that of the URL in the Web but extended to cover things other than Web pages). So an RDF description of a particular trial would consist of a set of triples of URIs, expressed as XML tags.

Ontologies

The final piece in the jigsaw is the creation of ontologies. The W3C proposals for the Semantic Web include the definition of a Web Ontology Language called OWL. OWL is a semantic mark-up language, an extension of RDF, which can be used to specify descriptions of things in the domain of interest: what are the general classes of entity that exist, what relationships are there between them, what properties or attributes can they have. In our example the ontology would have to include enough clinical knowledge to allow the search engine to match facts about a patient with facts about a trial: for example, that a trial of interventions for early-stage prostate cancer is not appropriate for a patient with a tumour greater than a certain size. The ontology will therefore have to include quite general facts about things like cancer, and specifically prostate cancer, and about tumours as well as about trials and patients. By providing tools that enable people to create and share ontologies, the W3C hopes to allow users, like the clinician in our example, to carry out automated reasoning on data provided by others – in our case the medical researcher.

Ontologies in health informatics

The development of sharable ontologies is perhaps the most important step along the way to the Semantic Web. Ontologies are also important in other contexts. In fact, any application where the developers need to think about the representation of the facts and relationships in a domain must be based on the kind of thinking that is formalised in an ontology. The motivation behind building explicit ontologies is often that people want the work that has to be put into analysing and understanding the domain to be cast in a form that others can use. Ontologies are sometimes said to be a mechanism for knowledge sharing and reuse. These days the sharing is very often a matter of creating a community of users, of building support for a proposed standard. Standards such as the Digital Imaging Communication (DICOM) and Health Level 7 (HL7), which is a set of standards for the interoperability of health care systems, are based on reference models that can be viewed as ontologies. We will discuss both of these in Chapter 9.

The more sophisticated terminology systems such as SNOMED CT are derived from clinical models, also known as ontologies. One of the themes of Chapter 7 was that simple enumerative coding schemes have proved unable to support the more complex applications that require standard terminologies, hence the drive to create systems such as SNOMED CT. It is because SNOMED CT provides not just a hierarchy of terms but also sets of criteria that define the meaning of those terms that it is an ontology of clinical concepts rather than simply a terminological standard. Later in this chapter we will talk about GALEN, an approach to terminology that is based on a very sophisticated approach to ontologies.

Projects such as openEHR, the electronic health records (EHR) architecture, and the various guideline representation formalisms can also be viewed as creating ontologies. We will look in more detail at some of these projects later in the chapter. First, we look at a short example of an ontology.

Building an ontology

Let us consider how we could use a language like OWL to represent the ontology or ontologies that would be required to support the application introduced above, in which the software tool was used to search the Semantic Web for clinical trials that might be appropriate for a particular patient. It would not be appropriate to present a detailed introduction to OWL here (see the W3C website for a good one[4]). Although RDF is expressed in XML and the syntax of XML is very simple, RDF statements are not as easy to read as one might wish and the problem is compounded when RDF is used to create an OWL ontology. However, the basic ideas that OWL makes use of are very simple. An OWL ontology consists of statements about classes of thing, statements about the properties that define the classes and statements about the things themselves. These statements are similar to the definitions of relations that we met in Chapter 6, under the heading Predicate Logic.

Classes

Classes are an abstraction mechanism; they group together things with similar characteristics. The set of individuals grouped together in a class, the instances of the class, is called the extension of the class. The set of characteristics that we associate with a class is called the intension. We sometimes say that a class can have an extensional or an intensional definition. Defining a class by its extension is a matter of enumerating the members. For example, the class of continents is defined as Europe, North America, South America, Africa, Asia, Australasia and Antarctica. The list of members is the definition. Defining a class by its intension is a matter of asserting criteria that can be used to distinguish members of the class from non-members.

Classes in OWL can be defined extensionally or intensionally. An extensional definition is provided when we describe a class by enumerating the instances of the class. An intensional definition is provided when we specify a property restriction for the class, that is to say when we specify a range of values for some property that class members can have. We can also create classes out of other classes: for example, defining a class as the intersection of two other classes, or as the union of two classes or as the complement of a class.

The formalism is slightly more complicated than this account would suggest since in OWL we have to distinguish between statements that *describe* a class and statements that *define* a class. We can create a class *description* by enumerating all the members of the class, by specifying a range of values for some property that members have or by one of the three operations on classes (intersection, union and complement). These class descriptions are then used to create the axioms that *define* classes. Class axioms associate descriptions with named classes. In OWL we first name a class, and then define it by creating axioms from class descriptions. An axiom can associate a class description with a named class in one of three ways. An axiom can state that a class description is:

- a necessary condition for membership of the named class (the description is of a subclass of the named class);
- a sufficient condition for membership (the description is of an equivalent class to the named class);
- an excluding condition (the description is the complement of the named class).

So, for example, we could create named classes by asserting the existence of the classes Human, Gender, Women, Mother. We could assert axioms to define the classes as follows:

- **Gender** is *equivalent* to the class description *enumerated* as **male** and **female**.

- **Women** is *equivalent* to the class description that is an *intersection* of the class **Human** and the class of things that have a *value* **female** for the *property* **has Gender**.
- **Mother** is *equivalent* to the class description that is an *intersection* of the class **Women** and the class of things that have a *value* **greater than 1** for the *property* **has number of children**.

Properties

In thinking about ontologies, it helps to make a clear separation between the statements that describe the classes and those that describe instances of the classes. Both will include statements about properties. In OWL, however, classes do not actually have properties. It is the instances that have the properties. So when we make a statement about a property in the description of a class, it is to say something about the range of values that instances of the class can have for a particular property. This can either be a statement of a property restriction, which, as explained above, serves as part of the definition of the class, or it can simply be a statement about the kind of thing the property is. So, for example, there might be a property restriction for the class 'paediatric patients', which says that the value of property 'age' is less than 18. Another statement, which could be associated with the class 'patient', might simply say that the values of the property 'age' are normally expressed as integers.

OWL distinguishes between properties (such as age) that link instances to datatypes (such as integers) and properties that link instances to other instances. So, for example, a property of the class 'patient' could link to the patient's normal GP, where GP would be another class in the ontology.

Statements about the properties of particular instances take the form of triples. We assert that a particular instance (e.g. a patient) has a particular value for some property. So, patient John Smith has age 46, for example. John Smith is a patient of Dr Jones, for another example.

OWL allows users to specify a number of features of properties, and indeed to create hierarchies of properties that are specialisations of other properties. Users can specify that values for a property must be members of a particular class description.

Individuals

Finally, individuals are defined with individual axioms that assert facts about class membership and property values of individuals and also facts about individual identity. Questions of identity are of crucial importance for ontologies that are designed to be shared across the Web, since it is not practical to assume that a single convention is used to name all of the instances of all the classes. In this account I am glossing over a number of special features of OWL and RDF to do with the management of what are called namespaces, essentially sets of unique identifiers for instances, properties and classes. Importantly, OWL reasoners cannot assume that two instances with different names are actually distinct entities. It is because this cannot in general be assumed that OWL allows you to specify that it is the case that instance A and instance B are different things.

An example

Consider the trial summary presented in Box 8.1. This is an edited version of a real trial summary published on www.clinicaltrials.gov, a website supported by the US government through the NIM. One way of viewing the format of the summary would be as the assertion of a set of values for the following properties of clinical trials:

- title;
- purpose;
- procedure;
- study type;
- study design;
- inclusion criteria;
- exclusion criteria;
- expected total enrollment;
- contact information;
- study start date;

We could define a class 'clinical trials' and assert these properties for instances of the class. We might use a restriction on the values that study design could take to define subclasses of trials with particular designs: blinded, randomised and so forth. However, a taxonomy of clinical trials would probably have a rather flat hierarchy. Most of the information one might want to record will be about specific trials, it will be about instances rather than classes.

One major difficulty in thinking about the 'clinical trials' class is working out how to represent the values for the properties. The properties 'title' and 'purpose' can perhaps be asserted as datatype properties having the value 'string' since we may not need to store anything other than 'canned text' when we assert these properties for specific instances of clinical trials. The possible values of 'study type' and 'study design' could be enumerated. The 'contact information' property is important since addresses are structured pieces of information and ones found in many different contexts, so we may want to define a datatype or a class for 'addresses'. The 'study start date' could be a defined type handling dates and 'expected total enrollment' will be an integer.

The most difficult issue concerns the inclusion and exclusion criteria. The simplest thing would be to assert that they are simply datatype properties having the datatype 'string'. However, we want to support applications that can reason about the suitability of patients for trials. We therefore need to represent the underlying logic and the clinical content of inclusion and exclusion criteria in terms that can automatically be matched against descriptions of patients. We will need to have recourse to something like SNOMED CT in order to do this, since the descriptions will be created by other applications.

Box 8.1 A summary of a clinical trial

Title: Propranolol for Syncope with Sympathoadrenal Imbalance

Purpose: This study will examine the effectiveness of the drug propranolol in preventing fainting in patients with sympathoadrenal imbalance (SAI). SAI is a particular pattern of nervous system and chemical responses in which the blood vessels in skeletal muscles do not remain constricted appropriately during standing for a long time. This can lower blood pressure and cause fainting.

Procedure: Patients enrolled in the study take propranolol pills in increasing doses during the first week of the study to determine the proper dose for the individual. Then, the drug is stopped until the experimental phase of the study begins. In this phase, patients are randomly assigned to take either propranolol or placebo for four days. On the fourth day, the patient undergoes a test in which the patient remains upright for 45 minutes while blood pressure, heart rate, blood flows, skin electrical conduction and electrocardiogram (ECG) are measured. The test procedure is repeated after one week. Patients who were given propranolol for the first session take a placebo for the repeat session, and those who were given placebo take propranolol.

Study type: Interventional

Study Design: Treatment

Inclusion criteria: Subjects are patients referred for evaluation of chronic orthostatic intolerance.
   Patients enter into the trial after they are determined to have SAI.

Exclusion criteria: Minors younger than 18 years are excluded.
   A candidate subject is excluded if there is a history of asthma or chronic obstructive pulmonary disease requiring bronchodilators, hepatic or renal failure, atrioventricular block of any degree, bradycardia, symptomatic congestive heart failure, severe anemia, psychosis, refractory ventricular arrhythmias, symptomatic coronary heart disease, insulin-dependent diabetes mellitus.
   Patients with known or suspected allergy or hypersensitivity to propranolol are excluded.
   Patients who must take medications daily in the following categories are excluded: anticoagulants, tricyclic antidepressants, barbiturates, aspirin, acetaminophen, insulin, bronchodilators.
   Pregnant or lactating women are excluded.

Expected total enrollment: 24

Contact information: National Institute of Neurological Disorders and Stroke, 9000 Rockville Pike, Bethesda, MD, 20892, USA

Study start date: 9 May 2003

One way of representing the required information about the inclusion and exclusion criteria would be to define a subclass of the class 'patient', the subclass being the set of patients who would be eligible for the propranolol trial. We can then use the OWL syntax for necessary and sufficient conditions to set out the property restrictions associated with both the inclusion and exclusion criteria. Reasoning using the ontology would then be a matter of ascertaining whether a given patient could be classified in the subclass 'patients eligible for the propranolol trial'. Table 8.1 sets out how such a class might be defined in an OWL-like syntax. The first five statements are a set of necessary criteria for members of the class 'eligible patients'. Each has the form:

Eligible patients is a subclass of X,

where X is not a named class but a criterion or set of criteria. For example, in the fifth statement X is the criterion 'complement of property restriction: property pregnant has value true'. This criterion defines a set, the set of non-pregnant people, being the complement of the set of pregnant people. An instance can only be a member of the set of 'eligible patients' if it is also a

Table 8.1 An OWL-like definition of the class 'eligible patients', instances of which will be the patients eligible for inclusion in the trial summarised in Box 8.1.

Eligible patients is a subclass of
  intersection of
    class of patients
    property restriction: property diagnosis has value SAI
Eligible patients is a subclass of
  complement of
    property restriction: property age has value <18
Eligible patients is a subclass of
  complement of
    property restriction: property diagnosis has value excluded condition
Eligible patients is a subclass of
  complement of
    property restriction: property current medication has value excluded medication
Eligible patients is a subclass of
  complement of
    property restriction: property pregnant has value true
Excluded condition is equivalent to
  enumeration of
    asthma, obstructive pulmonary disease, renal failure, atrioventricular block,
    bradycardia, symptomatic congestive heart failure, severe anaemia, psychosis, refractory
    ventricular arrhythmias, symptomatic coronary heart disease, insulin-dependent diabetes
    mellitus, allergy to propranolol
Excluded medication is equivalent to
  enumeration of
    anticoagulants, tricyclic antidepressants, barbiturates, aspirin, acetaminophen, insulin,
    bronchodilators

member of this set, and of those in the other four statements. Since most of the criteria in the description of the trial are exclusion criteria, most of the definitions involve the 'complement' criterion. The third and fourth statements contain criteria that relate to defined classes: the set of 'excluded conditions' and the set of 'excluded medications'. Both of these are defined, in the sixth and seventh statements, through the enumeration of the instances that make up the classes.

Note that the names given to the classes in Table 8.1 – 'eligible patients', 'excluded conditions' and 'excluded medications' – would not be sufficiently precise in a system that was intended to deal with multiple trials. A more sophisticated approach would be required that either explicitly or otherwise incorporated the name of the trial into the class name.

Description logics

Ontologies set out like this are sometimes referred to as description logics (although some of the detail passed over in this account of RDF means that OWL cannot be treated straightforwardly as a description logic)[5]. One of the characteristics of a description logic is that there is a separation between what is termed taxonomic knowledge (the T-Box) and assertional knowledge (the A-Box). Knowledge about how classes are defined is taxonomic knowledge; it introduces the vocabulary that is to be used to describe the domain. The OWL assertions that describe classes and set out the necessary and sufficient criteria for class membership constitute the T-Box. The A-Box, in contrast, consists of the assertions about the individuals that make up the classes.

Reasoning with description logics

The essence of taxonomic (T-Box) reasoning is subsumption; that is, identifying whether the definition of one class subsumes another. It is analogous to the notion of implication introduced in the discussion of logic in Chapter 6, in that just as we said that A implies B meant that if A is true, then B must be true, so if A is subsumed by (is a subset of) B then if something is a member of A, then it must be a member of B. The operators we use in logic (implies, and, or, not) all have their equivalents in what is called Set Theory (subsumption, intersection, union, complement) that allow reasoning about the membership of classes. In this application, however, we are reasoning with the T-Box *and* the A-Box, since we want to establish whether instances of the class of patients are members of a particular subclass: the subclass 'patients eligible for the propranolol trial'.

Modelling health care

Ontologies are developed in health care for a variety of applications. The following sections present three different attempts to build a model of a domain within health care. They differ in the extent to which the developers are committed to the idea of 'reusable knowledge' or sharable ontologies and in the extent to which the approach to modelling resembles that taken in the example above. All are significant real-world projects, however, involving substantial commitments from large groups of collaborators.

GALEN

GALEN is one of the best known attempts to develop an explicit model of clinical concepts[6]. The project, which has been led by Alan Rector *et al.* at the University of Manchester since the early 1990s, has produced a modelling language known as GRAIL (GALEN representation and integration language), a common reference model of clinical concepts, a drug ontology for use in GP prescribing systems and an open-source community, openGALEN. Although a detailed account of GRAIL would be beyond the scope of this book, its approach is based on a description logic, and the summary given above of OWL should provide the interested reader with some of the necessary theoretical background.

Untangling hierarchies

The authors of GALEN have identified a set of principles that they believe must be respected in the design of ontologies. The aim is to avoid the 'tangling' of hierarchies that occurs in many of the systems described in Chapter 7. Consider, for example, the way in which burns are classified in CTV3. There is a concept *burn* with 14 different subcategories, one of which is *burn of skin of body region* (another is *thermal burn – disorder* and the other 12 have the form *burn of X* where *X* is *eye structure, ear structure*, etc.). The concept *burn of skin of body region* has two subcategories: *burn of skin* and *burns as a percentage of body surface involved*. The second of these has subcategories for *less than 10% of body surface involved, 10–19% of body surface involved*, and so on. The subcategories of *burn of skin* include four that identify body regions and two others: *sunburn* and *superficial friction burn*. The burns of lower limb, to take an example of a subcategory of *burns of skin*, are further classified by region and then by extent; for example, one can end up with *full thickness burn of thigh*. Elsewhere in CTV3 there is an optional code for *accident due to contact with hot or corrosive substance*, which has numerous subcategories including *cigarette burn* and, bizarrely, *doughnut burn*.

Looking at the classification, shown in Table 8.2, it is obvious that different attributes of burns are being used to make the classification (location, structure affected, cause, extent, severity) but that the classification is neither complete nor logical. When I say that it is not complete, I mean that the ideas used in the classification could generate a much larger set of possibilities, including, for example, *sunburn of lower limb covering less than 10% of the body's surface*. When I say that the classification is not logical, I mean that, for example, it seems wrong that *thermal burn* is an alternative to *burn of skin of body region*, or that *burn of skin* is a subcategory of *burn of skin of body region*, or

Table 8.2 Part of the Read Codes Version 3 concept hierarchy showing a selection of the terms available for the classification of burns.

Burn
Thermal burn disorder
Burn of ear structure
Burn of eye structure
...
Burn of skin of body region
Burn of skin
Burn of head, face, neck
Burn of upper limb
Burn of trunk
Burn of lower limb
Burn of buttock
Burn of hip
Burn of thigh
Superficial burn of thigh
Partial thickness burn of thigh
Full thickness burn of thigh
Burn of knee
Burn of lower leg
Burn of ankle and foot
Multiple burn of lower limb
Superficial burn of leg
Partial thickness burn of leg
Full thickness burn of leg
Sunburn
Superficial friction burn
Burns as a percentage of body surface involved

that *superficial friction burn* should occur at the same level in the hierarchy as *burn of lower limb*.

The approach taken in GALEN is to specify a concept *burn lesion* and not to specify any more specific concepts but to specify a set of properties for burns that can be used to create definitions of more restricted classes of burns. So GALEN allows statements such as:

> *Burn lesion which*
>   *has Location Arm*
>   *has Depth half Thickness*
>   *has Extent 4 cm²*
>   *has Circumstances Kitchen Accident*
>   *has Cause Heat*

The idea is that all the different ways in which burns can be classified – by location, depth, extent, circumstances and cause – are separated out and, rather than being used to specify different subclasses within a single tangled

Table 8.3 Part of the GALEN taxonomy derived by composition and classification.

BurnLesion *which* hasCause Chemical
    BurnLesion *which* <hasCause Chemical hasLocation UpperExtremity>
      BurnLesion *which* <hasCause Chemical hasLocation Hand>
        BurnLesion *which* <hasCause Chemical hasLocation PalmarSurfaceOfHand>
        ...

   ...

 BurnLesion *which* hasCause Acid
  BurnLesion *which* <hasCause Acid hasLocation UpperExtremity>
    BurnLesion *which* <hasCause Acid hasLocation Hand>
      BurnLesion *which* <hasCause Acid hasLocation PalmarSurfaceOfHand>
      ...

  ...

 BurnLesion *which* hasCause Alkali
  ...

 ...

 ...

BurnLesion *which* hasCause Heat
  BurnLesion *which* hasCause Heat
    BurnLesion *which* <hasCause Heat hasLocation UpperExtremity>
      BurnLesion *which* <hasCause Heat hasLocation Hand>
        BurnLesion *which* <hasCause Heat hasLocation PalmarSurfaceOfHand>

 ...

 ...

hierarchy defined in advance, can be used to generate distinct, orthogonal taxonomies. In CTV3 burns are first classified either by cause (if they are given one of the codes for accidents) or by location or by extent, and if classified by location, they are next classified either by sublocation or cause (sunburn or friction burn) and then by depth. In GALEN, the description logic can be used to specify increasingly specific categories of burn by adding descriptors in whatever order suits a particular application, as shown in Table 8.3.

The GALEN drug ontology

The first task in building a taxonomy of this kind is therefore to identify the set of axes to be used in classification. In the drug ontology, drugs are classified according to their ingredients, form and route, pharmacological action, physiological action, indications, side-effects, interactions, contraindications and pharmacodynamics[7]. The high-level structure of the ontology is presented in Figure 8.1 and a fragment of the resulting ontology is shown in Table 8.4. The structure is designed in order to provide a convenient mechanism for representing the domain, in this case drugs as described in the British National Formulary. The ontology was developed for a specific purpose: to support a GP prescribing system, but the intention was that

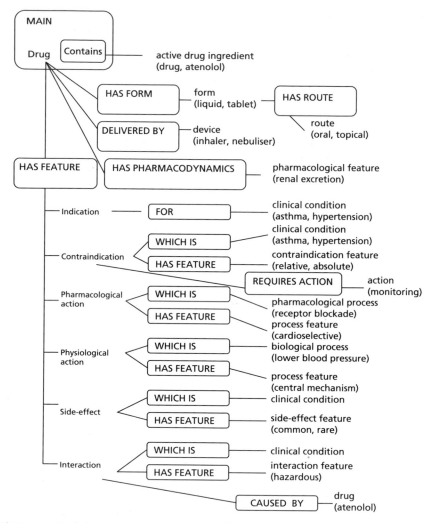

Figure 8.1 High-level structure of the GALEN drug ontology. From [7] with permission. © 1999 Elsevier.

representation should not be determined by the needs of that application, and should be completely reusable.

The authors claim that untangling the hierarchy of drugs made the representation of the domain relatively simple, despite the fact that standards bodies had previously failed in several attempts to determine a rational classification of forms, routes and preparations for drugs. The success of this project seems to serve as a demonstration of the promise of the approach; the real test, however, will come when someone attempts to reuse the ontology in a new and different application.

Table 8.4 A fragment of the GALEN drug ontology describing propranolol. This drug is considered prototypical and is therefore defined as an 'index drug'. Specific beta blockers will inherit contraindications defined for this class. The drug is delivered systemically and blocks beta adrenoceptors.

MAIN drug
HAS FORM ROUTE systemic
HAS DRUG FEATURE pharmacological action
  WHICH IS blockade
    ACTS ON beta adrenoceptor
HAS DRUG FEATURE information source
  IS PART OF contraindication index drug
PROPERTIES
  HAS DRUG FEATURE absolute contraindication
    WHICH IS personal history
      IS HISTORY OF obstructive airways disease

OpenEHR

One of the principle aims of health informatics has been the development of electronic patient record systems. Patients' notes are often stored on computers, but relatively few are stored in a way that allows sophisticated processing of the information. For example, a common goal is to allow the merger of information from different providers to create a single cradle-to-grave record of a patient's care. Information in such a record would have to be represented in a way that allowed different users to access information of different kinds in different ways. An ITU nurse will want access to detailed information about the patient's state over a short period; the patient's GP will require very different information about the stay in the ITU.

One initiative that is supporting the development of such 'systems of systems' is openEHR, pronounced 'open air'[8]. This is an open-source collaboration developing an information model for EHRs. Unlike GALEN, the resulting model is not concerned with clinical terms, but rather with the structure of medical records. The openEHR model consists of two main elements: a reference information model and a set of archetypes and templates. The reference model defines the various entities that are used to structure clinical records, and deals with concepts such as 'folders and compositions'. Archetypes are descriptions of valid entries expressed in a formal manner, which enables them to be shared between systems. For example, a blood pressure archetype represents a description of all the information a clinician might want to report about a blood pressure measurement. The openEHR foundation has produced a knowledge representation formalism, known as the archetype definition language (ADL) to help interested parties develop archetypes[9].

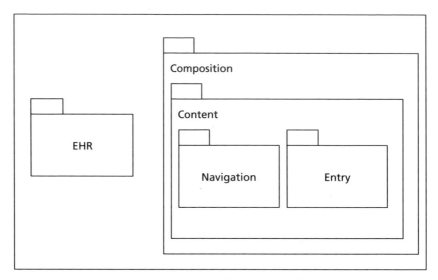

Figure 8.2 An overview of the openEHR information model.

The openEHR information model

In openEHR parlance, an EHR consists of a set of compositions. Compositions are the top-level 'data container' in the record, as shown in Figure 8.2. They are used to record both information about events and also what are termed 'persistent' data items, things such as the patient's family and social history, the problem list, current medications, therapeutic precautions, vaccination history, lifestyle and active care plans. The content of a composition consists of a 'navigation' and an 'entry'. The navigation part provides the structure used to organise information in the record. The structure is provided through a system of folders. Each patient's record consists of a set of folders. Each folder refers to a set of compositions. The entries contain all information that is to be recorded, as observations, evaluations or instructions. The model is highly abstract; it deals not with the specifics of a particular patient's record, nor indeed with any clinical content but rather provides a conceptual model of what a patient record is.

Archetypes in openEHR

The openEHR foundation defines archetypes as models of domain concepts. Their primary purpose in openEHR is to provide a way of managing generic data so that it conforms to domain structures and constraints. The definition of an archetype, in the openEHR ADL, has two elements: the constraint definition and the data definition, shown in Figure 8.3. Recall that in a description logic there are two elements: the T-Box that contains taxonomic knowledge and the A-Box that contains assertional knowledge. The distinction here is similar. The constraint definition is rather like the property

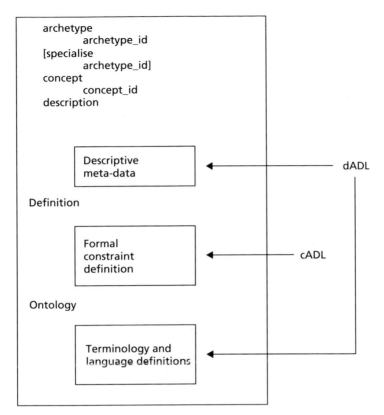

Figure 8.3 The constraint definition and the data definition for an openEHR archetype.

restrictions used to define classes in OWL. The data definition syntax provides a mechanism for expressing instance data.

NHS Health Care Modelling Programme

In the 1980s, the NHS attempted to define a comprehensive standard data model for all NHS computing applications. In one project, the Korner Steering Group developed a set of 'minimum data-sets' for various areas of NHS activity. They defined the minimum information that had to be collected on a regular basis to allow effective management of the service. This led to what was known as the HCHS minimum data-set model, which in turn was replaced by the *NHS Data Dictionary*, which is still in use today. It defines a standard for the recording of NHS data for administrative purposes[10].

Another project, initiated around the same time as the Korner report, led to what was known as the common basic specification (CBS)[11]. This developed a generic conceptual model of the activity of health care delivery. It was intended to ensure the integrity of an NHS data model that would go further than the minimum data-set, and support clinical care, not just administration. In essence, it was an attempt to define an ontology for the processes involved in health care. The CBS programme, which ran for about 5 years, worked with about 30 mostly pre-existing IT projects, and examined business areas across the health service. The CBS generic model was published in 1992, then reworked and republished as a series of application views in 1993. An assessment board looking at the outcomes of the project came to a favourable conclusion and in 1995 the programme was re-invented as the NHS Health Care Modelling Programme with a mission 'to extend and maintain models and modelling techniques that could be used by the NHS to help ensure the coherence and completeness of central information management initiatives'. Information about the programme could, until recently, be found on a website, the front page for which was last modified in 2000 and which was clearly marked as 'archived' and 'no longer supported'. At the time of writing it seems no longer to be accessible.

The CBS is large and complex. The 'Provide Patient Care' view of the model consists of 26 diagrams covering notions such as 'Establish Basis for Care', 'Assemble Patient Evidence', 'Interpret Patient Information', 'Agree Objectives for Care'. CBS was used, apparently successfully, in the development of a hospital information system for an acute Trust. Of course CBS cost millions to develop, took years to design and was intended to be generic, so if it was used once and once only, the project must be considered to have failed. The whole point of an ontology like this is that you use it more than once.

It was not developed by vendors, nor, crucially, was it developed in order to solve a problem that the purchasers of hospital systems perceived as important. It might, arguably, have been in the best interests of the NHS to ensure that all Trusts bought systems that were designed using a CBS, but it was not in the best interests of any individual Trust to require that their supplier adopted the specification. It might have been adopted if the NHS nationally had decided to require that Trusts purchase systems developed using the CBS, but that would have been a difficult and unpopular position to adopt. It would, for example, have prevented Trusts from buying cheap 'off-the-shelf' systems from suppliers serving other international markets, significantly the US market.

In recent years the process by which hospital systems are procured has changed[12]. The government has instituted a National Programme for IT, which insists that procurement is done centrally, with large regions signing contracts, each with a single supplier, often a consortium. The supplier contracts to supply not a system but rather the services that the system makes possible, over the lifetime of the contract. The risk involved in making the project work remains with the supplier and is not passed on to the purchaser. There is a process of, quite determined, standardisation involved. It is exactly the kind of process that was not around at the time CBS was developed, and it reflects a determination that the NHS should exploit its sheer size and purchasing power when dealing with suppliers. As a result, different Trusts will end up being provided with similar systems but the standardisation will not be driven by the same process that lay behind CBS; it will be closer to the process by which Microsoft Word became a standard format for the exchange of electronic documents. Instead of the NHS deciding on an all-encompassing underlying model to ensure that diverse systems are compatible, which was the idea behind CBS, it has taken a strategic decision forcing the different parts of the organisation to buy, pretty much, the exact same product.

Ontologies and standards

Each of the ontologies reviewed in this chapter, and each of the terminologies discussed in the previous one, could be considered an attempt to define a standard. The issue of standards is of enormous importance to health informatics. In Chapter 9 we consider two attempts to define standards in health informatics. They differ from the initiatives described in this chapter because they are concerned less with how health care or clinical concepts can be represented and more with what must be specified to allow different clinical systems to cooperate.

References

1. Sowa J. *Knowledge Representation: Logical, Philosophical and Computational Foundations*. Pacific Grove, CA: Brooks/Cole, 2000.
2. Naughton J. *A Brief History of the Future*. London: Phoenix, 2000.
3. Berners-Lee T, Hendler J, Lassila O. The Semantic Web. *Sci Am* May 2001. http://www.sciam.com
4. McGuiness D, van Harmelen F. *OWL Web Ontology Language Overview*. http://www.w3.org/TR/2004/REC-owl-features-20040210/ (accessed 12 February 2004).
5. Baader F *et al.* (eds) *The Description Logic Handbook: Theory, Implementation and Applications*. New York: Cambridge University Press, 2003.
6. Rector AL, Rogers JE, Zanstra PE, Van Der Haring E. OpenGALEN: pen-source medical terminology and tools. *Proc AMIA Symp* 2003;982.
7. Solomon WD, Wroe CJ, Rector AL, Rogers JE, Fistein JL, Johnson P. *A Reference Terminology for Drugs*. Annual Fall Symposium of American Medical Informatics Association, Washington DC. Philadelphia, PA: Hanley & Belfus, 152–155: 1999.
8. OpenEHR Foundation. *Introducing openEHR*. http://www.openehr.org/ (accessed 25 May 2005).
9. Beale T, Heard S (eds). *Archetype Definition Language*. http://www.openehr.org/ (accessed 25 May 2005).
10. NHS Data Model and Dictionary Service. *NHS Data Dictionary Version 3*. http://www.nhsia.nhs.uk/datastandards/pages/dd/index.asp (accessed 25 May 2005).

11. Harris J. The NHS common basic specification: why top-level ontologies don't work. www.virtualtravelog.net/entries/2004/01/ (accessed 25 May 2005).
12. Humber M. National programme for information technology. *BMJ* 2004; 328(7449):1145–1146.

CHAPTER 9

Standards in health informatics

This chapter deals with a similar theme to the last, but focuses on just two initiatives that have an enormous impact on the design and implementation of computer systems for applications in health care. These are two widely accepted standards. Both are based on an underlying model that is represented, using the kinds of techniques discussed in Chapter 8, as an ontology.

HL7

One of the aims of standards in software is to allow different applications on different machines to work together, to become interoperable. The International Standards Organization (ISO) specifies a set of levels for Open Systems Interconnection (OSI), and these levels provide a measure of the degree of integration that a particular standard seeks to enable. The highest is level 7: the application level. Level 7 addresses such issues as definition of the data to be exchanged, security checks, participant identification and data exchange structuring. One of the most ambitious sets of health care standards is being developed by an organisation known as the Health Level 7 (HL7)[1]. HL7 is developing a range of standards for a variety of applications but is best known for work on messaging standards – standards that define the format of messages to be passed between different clinical systems, to allow the sharing of data. Figure 9.1 shows a fragment of an HL7 message, presented in XML.

At the heart of the HL7 methodology is a model of health care information known as the Reference Information Model (RIM)[2]. This is an attempt to describe the people and processes involved in health care at a level of abstraction that is appropriate for the specification of messaging standards.

The Reference Information Model

The HL7 RIM is set out using the unified modelling language (UML)[3]. UML was not developed specifically for health care or for knowledge representation. It was developed as a part of what computer scientists call 'object-oriented methodology'. This is a quite general and widely used approach to the specification, design and development of computer systems. One element of UML is the construction of what are called 'class diagrams'. The RIM is presented, on the HL7 website, as a class diagram. Classes in UML are

```
<?xml version="1.0"?>
<!DOCTYPE Pt SYSTEM "admitexamp1.dtd" [ ]>
<Pt> <!-- 1 -->
        <id V="12345" AA="100.12.92.81.5.7" APN="MRN"/> <!-- 2, 3 -->
        <status V="L" S="HL7003" R="3.0"/> <!-- 2 -->
        <isAroleOfPersnAsPt> <!-- 4, 5 -->
                <adminvGendr V="M" S="HL7001" R="3.0" PN="Male"/> <!-- 4 -->
                <brthDttm V="19790924162403-0800"/> <!-- 4, 6 -->
                <phon> <!-- 4 -->
                        <_TEL ADR="tel:(358)555-1234" USE="PRN EMR"/> <!--7, 9 -->
                </phon> <!-- 4 -->
                <hasSetPrsnNameForPt> <!--4, 8 -->
                        <_PrsnNameForPt>
                                <nm>
                                        <G V="Irma" CLAS="R"/>
                                        <G V="Corine" CLAS="R"/>
                                        <F V="Jongeneel" CLAS="R M"/>
                                        <D V="-"/>
                                        <F V="de Haas" CLAS="R B"/>
                                </nm>
                                        <purpse V="L" S="HL7005" R="3.0"/>
                        </_PrsnNameForPt>
                </PtPrsnName> <!-- 4 -->
        </isAroleOfPersnAsPt> <!-- 2 -->
        <hasAprimryProvdrIHCP> <!-- 2 -->
                <phon>
                        <_TEL ADR="tel:(358)555-1234" USE="PRN EMR"/> <!-- 8 -->
                        <_TEL ADR="tel:(358)555-4321" USE="FAX"/> <!-- 8 -->
                </phon>
                <isRoleOfPersnAsIHCP>
                        <hasPrsnNameForIHCP>
                                <nm>
                                        <G V="Bubba" CLAS="R"/>
                                        <G V="Corine" CLAS="R"/>
                                        <F V="Jongeneel" CLAS="R M"/>
                                        <D V="-"/>
                                        <F V="de Haas" CLAS="R B"/>
                                </nm>
                        </hasPrsnNameForIHCP>
                </isRoleOfPersnAsIHCP>
        </hasAprimryProvdrIHCP>
        <isInvlvdInPtEncntr T="PtEncntr"> <!-- 2 -->
```

Figure 9.1 An example of an HL7 message presented using an XML syntax.

```
<idV="12345A23"AA="100.12.92.81.5.7"APN="EID"/>
<startDttmV="19990924162403-0800"/>
<statusV="L"/>
<hasAsPartcpntSetEncntrPractnr>
        <_EncntrPractnr>
                <partcptnTypV="ATT"/>
                <isPartcpntForIHCP>
                        <phon>
                                <_TELADR="tel:(358)555-1234"USE="PRNEMR"/>
                        </phon>
                        <hasPrsnNameForIHCP>
                                <nm>
                                        <GV="Bubba"CLAS="R"/>
                                        <GV="Corine"CLAS="R"/>
                                        <FV="Jongeneel"CLAS="RM"/>
                                        <DV="-"/>
                                        <FV="deHaas"CLAS="RB"/>
                                </nm>
                        </hasPrsnNameForIHCP>
                </isPartcpntForIHCP>
        </_EncntrPractnr>
        <_EncntrPractnr>
                <partcptnTypeV="CONS"/>
                <isPartcpntForIHCP>
                        <phon>
                                <_TELADR="tel:(358)555-1234"USE="PRNEMR"/>
                                <!--8-->
                        </phon>
                        <hasPrsnNameForIHCP>
                                <nm>
                                        <GV="Billy-Bob<"CLAS="R"/>
                                        <FV="deHaas"CLAS="RB"/>
                                </nm>
                        </hasPrsnNameForIHCP>
                </isPartcpntForIHCP>
        </_EncntrPractnr>
        </hasAsPartcpntSetEncntrPractnr>
    </isInvlvdInPtEncntr><!--2-->
 </Pt><!--1-->
```

Figure 9.1 (*continued*)

abstractions, just as they are in OWL. A class is defined as a name, a set of attributes and a set of operations. The attributes of a class are the properties that can be used to describe instances of the class. The operations of a class are the functions it performs. The RIM is a static model and does not define operations for classes, which means the information it does represent is similar to that which would be expressed in an OWL ontology. In UML, classes are connected by various kinds of links. The generalisation link connects subsets to supersets, the aggregation and composition links identity to other forms of decomposition while association links are used to indicate other relationships between classes.

The RIM defines six 'back-bone' classes:

- Act – the actions that are executed and must be documented;
- Participation – the context for an act: who performed it, where and for whom;
- Entity – the physical things and beings that are of interest to, and take part in, health care;
- Role – the roles entities play in health care acts;
- ActRelationship – the relationship between acts;
- RoleLink – the relationships between roles.

A class diagram for the six is shown in Figure 9.2 with some of the subclasses of the Act and Entity class presented in Figures 9.3 and 9.4.

Acts in HL7

Acts are at the centre of the RIM. Acts include clinical observations, assessments (including diagnoses), treatments, attending patients and editing and maintaining the record. Acts connect to Entities in their Roles through Participations and connect to other Acts through ActRelationships. Participations are the authors, performers and other responsible parties as well as subjects, beneficiaries, tools and material. Participations represent performance while Roles represent competence. An Entity is generally a physical object; the only exception being organisations, which have the essential characteristics of entities despite their somewhat virtual character. The Entity hierarchy also covers living subjects including human beings.

The Act class is intended to be used not just to record the history of what was done, but also statements about what was planned, ordered, requested and so on. HL7 statements are not simply assertions to be stored on a patient's record; they can also be messages that are sent in order to make things happen: issuing a prescription, ordering a test, booking a theatre slot. The Act class has an attribute moodCode, which distinguishes between various moods (modalities might be a better word) of acts. Consider an act of blood glucose observation. If the mood is recorded as DEFINITION, the statement would be a specification of how blood glucose is measured. In INTENT mood, the author expresses the intention that blood glucose should be observed. In REQUEST mood, the author requests a blood glucose measurement. In EVENT mood, the author states that blood glucose was

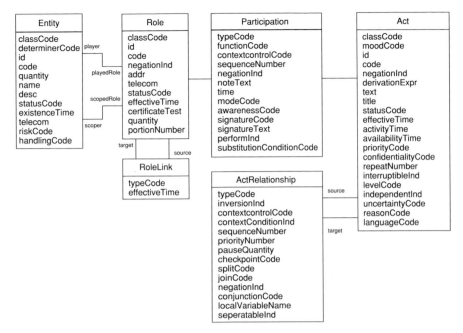

Figure 9.2 UML class diagram showing the back-bone classes of the HL7 Reference Information Model. From [1] with permission from Health Level Seven, Inc.

observed. In CRITERION mood, the author might define a target level for blood glucose.

It is worth looking in detail at what the HL7 documentation says about the definitions of one or two of the clinically significant subclasses of Acts.

An observation is defined in the HL7 documentation as an act of recognising and noting information about the subject, whose immediate and primary outcome is new data about a subject. Observations may simply be statements recording a clinician's assessment of findings or of the diagnosis but may equally well be a measurement or test result. The format allows for name-value-pairs but they will often have more complex structures, where the Observation includes a report of component observations.

A procedure is an act whose immediate and primary outcome is the alteration of the physical condition of the subject. Procedures may involve the disruption of some body surface (e.g. an incision in a surgical procedure) but would also include physiotherapy and even massage or acupuncture. The definition of procedure is slightly awkward, since it excludes many acts that are typically referred to as procedures, e.g. taking an X-ray, but includes such non-clinical things as such draining swamps (presumably relevant in accounts of public health campaigns). Many clinical activities combine Acts of Observation and Procedure nature into one composite. For instance, surgical procedures can include Observation steps. These are best represented by multiple component acts, each of the appropriate type.

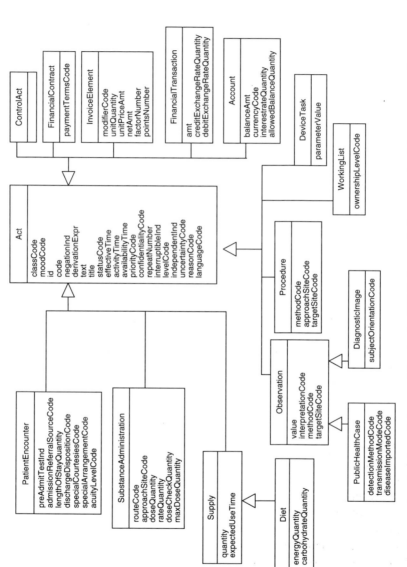

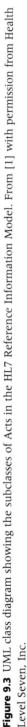

Figure 9.3 UML class diagram showing the subclasses of Acts in the HL7 Reference Information Model. From [1] with permission from Health Level Seven, Inc.

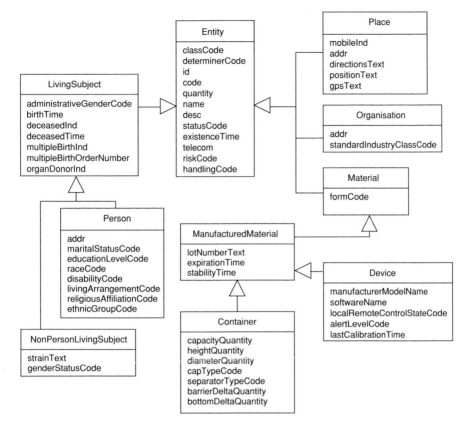

Figure 9.4 UML class diagram showing the subclasses of Entities in the HL7 Reference Information Model. From [1] with permission from Health Level Seven, Inc.

HL7 communications infrastructure

The classes outlined in Figures 9.2–9.4 are included in the RIM as part of an attempt to model clinical work and clinical processes, or at least to model as much of them as is necessary to support the work of HL7. The RIM also includes a number of other classes that are less to do with clinical processes and more to do with the technical detail of exchanging structured messages. There is a set of classes that define the communications infrastructure for HL7, including classes for message control such as:

- Acknowledgement
- Acknowledgement Detail
- Attention Line
- Batch
- Communication Function
- Message
- Transmission

Classes of query are also defined as well as document classes and a few others known as 'core infrastructure' that handle some technical limitations of the modelling.

HL7 methodology

The aim of HL7 is to define standards that allow IT systems to 'interoperate', that is, to respond to instructions and share data through the sending and receiving of messages. The role of the RIM is to support the development of diverse messaging standards by establishing a single 'reference model' for the information content of those messages. It is worth noting that the model presented in the RIM is not a model of the content of clinical concepts that are used in health care, in the sense that it does not talk about diseases or pathologies or the different kinds of drugs and treatments that there are. Rather it is a model of the kinds of acts and entities that health care systems deal in: of the 15 subclasses of acts defined in the RIM, 4 refer specifically to forms of financial transaction.

In Chapter 5, I made the point that interpreting data as information in-volved adopting a perspective. Different people would view the same data as containing different information depending on their perspective. Modelling a system, equally, requires that you take a perspective. A model, such as the RIM, is an abstraction, and abstracting means being selective, making choices about what to include and what to pass over. It is rather like creating a map. A cartographer's job is to depict just enough of a landscape to allow a useful representation to fit onto a folded sheet of paper, a small book or the inside back cover of a diary. He or she must select which features of the landscape to include and which to leave out. That selection, and this is the important point, will depend on the purpose for which the map is being made. The maps made for hikers differ from maps made for motorists. So the model developed to support the work of HL7 is very different to that which underpins GALEN or SNOMED CT. Whereas GALEN and SNOMED have clinical applications, HL7 is, essentially, concerned with standards for that part of the software industry that supplies organisations providing health care, so the content is less clinical and more administrative.

DICOM

A digital image is an array of data. A 512 × 512 pixel black-and-white image might consist of a sequence of 262 144 bytes of data, each byte representing a number between 0 and 255 to indicate the level of grey to be found at that point in the image. For this image to be displayed correctly, the software that puts it up on the screen must know that the 262 144 bytes represent a 512× 512 pixel and not a 256×1024 pixel image, that it is black and white rather than colour and that there is one byte of data per pixel. It must also know what convention is used to map from pixel values to grey levels, how the data are arranged and that there is data decompression or any other processing to be done before placing the image on the screen. All this information is generally stored in a section of data before the start of the actual image data, known as the header. Different image formats (jpeg, tiff, bmp, etc.) have different headers. Until the 1980s most digital medical images were created in file formats that were understood only by the device that created the image. However, a modern hospital radiology department wants to have a single system for storing, sharing and archiving medical images that will work with all of the imaging devices and all of the display workstations in the department, and indeed with those of other departments in the hospital, and with images acquired from machines in other hospitals, from which patients may have been transferred. That means being able to deal with images of different modalities (CT, MRI, PET, etc.) and images from machines made by different companies.

The American College of Radiology and the National Electrical Manufacturers Association first published a standard for medical image file formats in 1985[4]. The standard has now been almost universally adopted. Version 3 of the standard, now known as Digital Images and Communication in Medicine (DICOM), has also evolved so that it not only specifies an image file format that allows images created by one system to be read on another but also a network protocol allowing different imaging systems to communicate. It has also been extended further into the clinical world so the DICOM standard encompasses not just the information required to display an image correctly but also some of the information that a radiologist might record on making his or her assessment of the image.

Like HL7, which it is intended to complement, DICOM version 3 is presented as an object-oriented standard. The information model defines a set of object classes that provide an appropriate model of the domain, the world of medical imaging. The object classes are coupled with the service classes, which define the operations that must be performed on the data objects (these are the operations that must be performed in a networked imaging system, such as store, query and retrieve). Any two implementations of the set of service classes and information objects will be able to communicate effectively, to form a network.

In order to guarantee interoperability between machines while preserving the integrity of complicated clinical data, the standard has to be extraordinarily detailed. It is presented in 16 parts, the core elements of which are the information object definitions (IODs), the service class specifications and the data dictionary, totalling over a thousand pages in length.

Information object definitions

The DICOM model of the real world, the ontology if you like, is represented as a set of entity relationship diagrams, such as that shown in Figure 9.5. Each of the entities corresponds to an information object for which the standard provides an IOD. Each IOD specifies the set of attributes that describes and identifies instances of the object. So, for example, the patient IOD includes

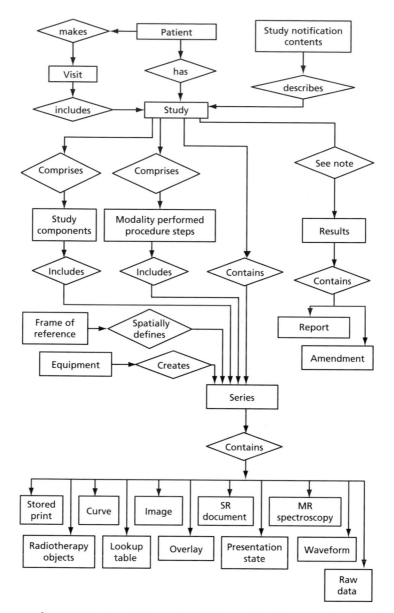

Figure 9.5 The DICOM view of the real world. From [1] with permission from Health Level Seven, Inc.

attributes such as patient name, patient ID, patient birth date, patient sex and so on.

Just as the information included in the HL7 RIM reflects the perspective of HL7 and concentrates on financial and administrative concerns, the DICOM model of the real world deals with the acquisition, storage and display of clinical images. The attributes listed in the different IODs contain a mixture of patient data and technical detail, specifying absolutely everything that is required for the correct display, interpretation and recording of a medical image. To illustrate the kind of information that is required, image pixel attributes include:

- Number of samples per pixel and their photometric interpretation. Monochrome images typically have one sample per image, and colour images generally have three. (Note: The commonest way of representing a colour image is by giving a separate pixel value for a red, green and blue image. Other representations are possible, for example, with one value for luminance and two 'chromacity' values.)
- Number of bits stored and allocated. If the acquisition device can resolve more than 2000 different levels of luminance, 12 bits would be wanted to store each pixel; however, the device might well allocate 16 bits, since dealing in whole bytes makes the memory management easier.
- Most significant bit. A holy war rages in computing between Big-Endians, who read multibyte registers from left to right, i.e. with the most significant, meaning largest, bit first, and Little-Endians, who read from right to left. On the one hand, Big-Endianism seems sensible because in English we read text from left to right; on the other hand, Little-Endianism is a more obvious way of storing numbers – if you think of the display on a digital calculator and count up from zero, the number in the display grows from right to left.
- Pixel aspect ratio. Not all pixels are square.

The DICOM standard distinguishes between composite and normalised object definitions. Earlier versions of the standard, developed before the object-oriented approach was adopted, grouped attributes together according to conventional usage rather than the structure of the real-world model. Patient name, for example, is given as an attribute of the image, because the patient name is conventionally stored with the image, whereas in the model it is clearly an attribute of the patient. In order to ensure backwards compatibility with previous versions, the current version of the standard includes normalised object definitions, which conform to the model, and composite object definitions – inherited from earlier versions – which contain attributes from more than one real-world object.

Service class specifications

Since DICOM is intended to allow imaging devices to be connected together and function via a network, the standard must not only define objects but a mechanism by which they can interoperate. This is done through the specification of service classes for use with the information objects. There are composite and normalised services for use with composite and normalised information objects.

Complex services are built out of service elements called DICOM message service elements, or DIMSEs. DIMSEs are classified as operations (e.g. 'store') or notifications (e.g. 'event report'). There are five DIMSEs (called DIMSE-C) for composite information objects and six (called DIMSE-N) for normalised information objects. The five DIMSE-C services are: C-Store, C-Get, C-Move, C-Find and C-Echo – these are all operations, as opposed to notification services. The DIMSE-N services include five operations: N-Get, N-Set, N-Action, N-Create and N-Delete, as well as one notification N-Event Report.

These DIMSEs are used to create service classes, defined in the DICOM standard, which perform the kinds of operations that imaging systems must perform, such as running queries, retrieving studies, printing images and so on.

Service object pairs

The functional unit of DICOM is the combination of an information object and a service class, a service–object pair, or SOP class. For example, the CT information object definition and the storage service class are combined to form the CT image storage SOP class. Each SOP class is assigned a unique identifier (UID), a series of numbers separated by points; the convention used here (that of the OSI or Open-Source Initiative) is a broader one than just DICOM, and all DICOM UIDs start with '1.2.840.10008'[5].

It is at the level of SOP classes that DICOM actually works, in the sense that when a manufacturer wishes to claim compliance with DICOM, it must produce a statement regarding which SOP classes are provided. Since the standard is, in part, about network functionality, applications can take one of two roles in respect of SOP classes; an application can be a service class user (SCU) or a service class provider (SCP). The distinction between an SCU and SCP is similar to that between a client and a server in a conventional network. To confirm that two DICOM devices are interoperable, you first identify all the activities for which the devices will have to exchange data, next which SOP classes will be required to support those activities and then check the device's DICOM conformance statements to ensure that the SOP classes are supported in the roles required. If one device is an SCU for a given class, the other must be an SCP.

Interoperability

To take a real world example, consider the DICOM conformance statement of the GE Senographe 2000D Full Field Digital Mammography machine[6]. This 102-page document includes, mercifully near the start, two tables, presented here as Table 9.1 and Table 9.2. One specifies the SOP classes for which the application entity (the Senographe 2000D) provides standard conformance as an SCU; the other specifies the SOP classes for which it provides standard conformance as an SCP.

The Senographe 2000D supports six SOP classes as an SCU and four as an SCP. The verification SOP class determines whether a DICOM application can

Table 9.1 According to the conformance statement of the GE Senographe 2000D, the application entity provides standard conformance to the above DICOM v3.0 SOP classes as an SCU.

SOP class name	SOP class UID
Digital mammography X-ray storage – for presentation	1.2.840.10008.5.1.4.1.1.1.2
Digital mammography X-ray storage – for processing	1.2.840.10008.5.1.4.1.1.1.2.1
Secondary capture image storage	1.2.840.10008.5.1.4.1.1.7
Study root query/retrieve information model – FIND	1.2.840.10008.5.1.4.1.2.2.1
Study root query/retrieve information model – MOVE	1.2.840.10008.5.1.4.1.2.2.2
Verification SOP class	1.2.840.10008.1.1

Table 9.2 According to the conformance statement of the GE Senographe 2000D, the application entity provides standard conformance to the above DICOM v3.0 SOP classes as an SCP.

SOP class name	SOP class UID
Digital mammography X-ray storage – for presentation	1.2.840.10008.5.1.4.1.1.1.2
Digital mammography X-ray storage – for processing	1.2.840.10008.5.1.4.1.1.1.2.1
Secondary capture image storage	1.2.840.10008.5.1.4.1.1.7
Verification SOP class	1.2.840.10008.1.1

be reached via the network. The SCU requests verification and the SCP responds. Three of the SOP classes supported are storage services for different IODs. When an SCU requests that an image be stored, it requests that the SCP receives the image. DICOM does not require that the SCP archives the image permanently, but merely that it accepts the image from the sender. The query/retrieve SOP provides two distinct services. With FIND, the SCU requests information about images and the SCP then responds with the requested information. With MOVE, the SCU asks that certain images be moved from the SCP either back to the SCU or elsewhere.

Now, say we want to use the Senographe 2000D with a given PACS implementation, say IDX's ImageCast[7]. Consider Table 9.3. We can see that if the proposed interaction requires that the PACS system displays digital mammograms, interoperability would seem to be supported. If the PACS system is required to handle the storage of digital mammograms, for processing, then there may be a problem.

Again, as with HL7, the view of the real world embodied in the DICOM models reflects the role of the standard. The aim is to allow purchasers to ensure that the devices they buy will function as part of a networked radiology department. The standard is not a model of radiology or of the work of a radiology department; it is closer to a description of software components at a level that is convenient for establishing interoperability.

Table **9.3** According to the conformance statement of the IDX ImageCast, the application entity provides standard conformance to the above DICOM v3.0 SOP classes as in the roles specified.

SOP class name	SOP class UID	Role
MR image storage	1.2.840.10008.5.1.4.1.1.4	SCU, SCP
Computed radiography image storage	1.2.840.10008.5.1.4.1.1.1	SCU, SCP
CT image storage	1.2.840.10008.5.1.4.1.1.2	SCU, SCP
Secondary capture image storage	1.2.840.10008.5.1.4.1.1.7	SCU, SCP
Ultrasound image storage	1.2.840.10008.5.1.4.1.1.6.1	SCU, SCP
Ultrasound multiframe image storage	1.2.840.10008.5.1.4.1.1.3.1	SCU, SCP
Nuclear medicine image storage	1.2.840.10008.5.1.4.1.1.20	SCU, SCP
X-ray angiographic image storage	1.2.840.10008.5.1.4.1.1.12.1	SCU, SCP
X-ray radiofluoroscopic image storage	1.2.840.10008.5.1.4.1.1.12.2	SCU, SCP
RT image storage	1.2.840.10008.5.1.4.1.1.481.1	SCU, SCP
Positron emission tomography image storage	1.2.840.10008.5.1.4.1.1.128	SCU, SCP
Digital X-ray image storage – for presentation	1.2.840.10008.5.1.4.1.1.1.1	SCU, SCP
Digital mammography image storage – for presentation	1.2.840.10008.5.1.4.1.1.1.2	SCU, SCP
Patient root query/retrieve information model – FIND	1.2.840.10008.5.1.4.1.2.1.1	SCU, SCP
Patient root query/retrieve information model – MOVE	1.2.840.10008.5.1.4.1.2.1.2	SCU, SCP
Study root query/retrieve information model – FIND	1.2.840.10008.5.1.4.1.2.2.1	SCU, SCP
Study root query/retrieve information model – MOVE	1.2.840.10008.5.1.4.1.2.2.2	SCU, SCP
Patient/study only root query/ retrieve information model – FIND	1.2.840.10008.5.1.4.1.2.3.1	SCU, SCP
SCU, SCP patient/study only root query/retrieve information mode – MOVE	1.2.840.10008.5.1.4.1.2.3.2	SCU, SCP
Verification	1.2.840.10008.1.1	SCU, SCP

Successful standards

Standards exist in many domains, not just in health care and not just in computing. Esperanto can be seen as an attempt to design a common standard for human communication. It does not seem to have been successful, and English is increasingly accepted as the standard international language. I am not quite sure why this is but it seems likely that the reasons are to do with the consequences of British imperialism or American economic dominance rather than to do with any inherent quality of the language that marks English out as being better than other candidates such as Esperanto, Latin or French. It is worth remembering that in a competitive market standards only succeed if individuals and organisations see that it is in their interests to comply. DICOM has been extremely successful because it was supported by the suppliers, who recognised that only by adopting such a standard could they meet the needs of their customers. Not all attempts to create standards for health care have been so successful.

Compare CBS or CTV3 to DICOM. Networked radiology departments need to ensure that they can use a single system to store and display images from different imaging devices. Real benefits accrue from the existence of a standard. It is because of these benefits that if a group of manufacturers can be persuaded to develop and adopt a standard, their products will have an added selling point. So, if it looks as though there is going to be a standard, everyone will want to adopt it. There are also significant benefits to be gained for a vendor from being closely involved in the development of the standard. No one wants to be forced, late in the game, to adopt someone else's standard having invested heavily in incompatible technology.

References

1. HL7. *Health Level 7*. http://www.hl7.org (accessed on 24 May 2005).
2. HL7. *HL7 Reference Information Model*. http://www.hl7.org (accessed on 24 May 2005).
3. Fowler M. *UML Distilled*. Reading, MA: Addison-Wesley, 2000.
4. ACR NEMA. *The DICOM Standard*. http://medical.nema.org/dicom/2004.html (accessed on 24 May 2005).
5. Open-Source Initiative. *The Open Source Initiative*. http://www.opensource.org/ (accessed on 24 May 2005).
6. GE Medical Systems Senographe 2000D. Acquisition Workstation Conformance Statement for DICOM v3.0. Technical Publications Direction 2246811–100, Revision 2 2000. General Electric Co.
7. IDX Imagecast. PACS Server 3.2 DICOM Conformance Statement 2004. IDX Systems Corporation.

CHAPTER 10
Probability and decision-making

In Chapter 5, I wrote that much of the work we do in health informatics is about building representations, and describing concepts and the relations between them. For a large class of health informatics applications the main challenge is to identify a structure that can provide the basis for forming database queries, making logical inferences, modelling software standards or whatever the application requires. There are, however, a host of other situations in which the analysis of the problem is a prelude to calculation: it is necessary to use the models together with some numerical statements and do some mathematical work to get any value out of the representation. Most of those applications will make use of some notion of probability.

Dealing with incomplete information

Say I toss a coin; what are the odds of it coming down heads? The answer is easy, although it can be stated in a number of ways: fifty-fifty, one in two, one to one, evens, 50% or 0.5. When I talk about probability I will use a number between 0 and 1, where 0 is absolute impossibility and 1 is absolute certainty. What exactly do we mean when we say that the probability of a coin coming down heads is 0.5? We mean that if we toss the coin several times, half the time it will come down heads. This is known as the *law of large numbers*[1]. If the number of events we observe is sufficiently large, the frequency of a given outcome is an accurate assessment of its probability. If we arrive at a measure of probability by measuring outcomes in this way, we can say that our measure is objective. It constitutes a fact about the frequency with which the outcome occurs.

We often want to talk about the likelihood of unique events, however, events for which there are no data on the frequency of possible outcomes. A physician might use the language of probability to express an assessment of the likelihood of a particular patient surviving an operation. This might be a quite subjective assessment, based on knowledge of the patient's particular circumstances rather than on statistics about the outcomes for previous patients. We can use the numbers we obtain from such subjective assessments in calculations just as we use objective assessments, but it is worth recognising that they are not exactly the same thing. It should also be remembered that interpreting subjective assessments of likelihood as probabilities is only one of a number of mathematical techniques for dealing with such quantitative assessments of belief.

We use probabilities to deal with the problem of incomplete information. If we knew everything there was to know about an event, we would not need to talk in terms of the probabilities of different outcomes because we would know what was going to happen. If we knew nothing about it, we could not even start to discuss the possible outcomes. It is only when we have incomplete information that we need to think about how we represent our degree of belief in a proposition. There are different ways in which information can be incomplete: it can be uncertain, in the way that information about the outcome of tossing a coin is uncertain. It can also be imprecise. If we are interested in quantifying the imprecision associated with a statement, rather than the probability of its being true, we might want to use fuzzy logic, which was discussed briefly in Chapter 6.

The next section sets out the axioms that describe how we deal, mathematically, with probabilities.

Axioms of probability

I use a notation in which the probability of some event having the outcome A is written $p(A)$. So we say that:

$0 \leq p(A) \leq 1$ *probability is a number between 0 and 1*

$p(\text{true}) = 1$ *absolute certainty has a value of 1.*

Further, we say that:

$p(A) + p(\text{not } A) = 1$ *the probability of an event occurring and the probability of it not occurring must add up to 1.*

These are axioms of probability. There are four such axioms, the three listed above and a fourth that needs a slightly more careful explanation.

Say I toss the coin twice, what is the probability of getting heads both times? One in four, or 0.25. We can work out the probability that two events both occur by multiplying together the probabilities for the two separate events: $0.5 \times 0.5 = 0.25$. At least we can work it out for coin tosses. It is not always that simple. Say I have 20 students, of whom 12 are male and 4 are bearded. The probability that a student picked at random will be male is $12/20 = 0.6$. The probability that a student picked at random will be bearded is $4/20 = 0.2$. Does it follow that the probability of a random student being male and bearded is 0.6×0.2? Well, no. When we combine probabilities, we must do so in a way that reflects the fact that some probabilities are related. Most bearded people are men. We have to multiply the probability of a randomly selected student being male (0.6) by the probability of him being bearded, given that he is male ($4/12 = 0.33$), which turns out to be 0.2. Since only male students are bearded, the probability of a student being male and bearded is just the probability of him being bearded.

Take another example. In my local bookmakers you can bet on the winner of Saturday's football match (event A). Especially bold punters are encouraged to bet that a particular player will score first (event B) and that his team will then go on to win. Clearly if an Arsenal player (say, Henry) scores the first goal, it becomes more likely that Arsenal will win the match. Working out the odds to offer for the combined bet (Henry scores first and Arsenal win), the bookmaker must combine the prior odds he would give for the two events in a way that reflects the fact that the two are related. He must multiply the probability of Henry's goal by the probability of Arsenal winning *given that Henry has scored*. In our notation we write $p(A, B)$ to denote the probability of A and B occurring, while we write $p(A|B)$ to denote the probability of A given B. And we say that:

$$p(A, B) = p(A|B) \times p(B).$$

This is the fourth axiom of probability. Note that if two events are independent (like coin tosses), then $p(A|B) = p(A)$ and the probability of the conjunction is just the product of the two probabilities.

We could just as easily have written this axiom with A and B the other way round:

$$p(A, B) = p(B|A) \times p(A),$$

from which it follows that:

$$p(A|B) \times p(B) = p(B|A) \times p(A),$$

and hence that:

$$p(A|B) = p(B|A) \times p(A)/p(B),$$

which some of you may recognise as Bayes' theorem[1]. To put it another way:

$$p(\text{disease}|\text{symptom}) = p(\text{symptom}|\text{disease}) \times p(\text{disease})/p(\text{symptom}).$$

The probability that a patient with symptom S has disease D is given by the probability of the symptom given the disease multiplied by the prior probability of the disease divided by the prior probability of the symptom.

Bayes' theorem and diagnostic tests

Let us look at an application of Bayes' theorem in interpreting the results of a diagnostic test, say a mammogram. A mammogram, or breast X-ray, is the diagnostic test used in screening for breast cancer. In any diagnostic test there are four possible outcomes, corresponding to the four cells of Table 10.1. The test may correctly identify a patient with the disease (a, true positive), correctly identify a patient without the disease (d, true negative), erroneously label a disease case as disease-free (c, false negative) or errone-

Table 10.1 The four possible outcomes of a diagnostic test.

	With disease	Without disease	Total
Test positive	a	b	a + b
Test negative	c	d	c + d
Total	a + c	b + d	

ously label a disease-free case as diseased (b, false positive). There are four different statistics commonly used to measure the accuracy of a test:
- Sensitivity, the proportion of disease cases correctly identified by the test $= a/(a + c)$
- Specificity, the proportion of disease-free cases correctly identified by the test $= d/(b + d)$
- Positive predictive value, the probability of a patient identified by the test having the disease $= a/(a + b)$
- Negative predictive value, the probability of a patient not identified by the test not having the disease $= d/(c + d)$

The sensitivity of a test tells us how good it is at picking up disease cases. The specificity of a test tells us how good it is at not picking up disease-free cases. Inevitably there is a trade-off between sensitivity and specificity. The more aggressive we are about trying to find every case of breast cancer that is out there, the more we will end up bringing in disease-free women. Let us see how the numbers stack up in a realistic example.

The predictive value of mammography

Imagine that mammography has a sensitivity of 77% and a specificity of 95%, and assume that the incidence of breast cancer in the screening population is 0.6%. If your mammogram is positive, how likely is it that you have breast cancer? You might think that, given that the test has a sensitivity of 77%, you are pretty likely to have cancer. It is not a complicated calculation but one that a lot of people have difficulty with. We do not seem to find it easy to deal with probabilities expressed as ratios of percentages[2]. Table 10.2, however, shows what the outcomes would be for a population of 10 000. An incidence of 0.6% would mean that in a population of 10 000 there would be 60 cases of cancer. A sensitivity of 77% would mean that out of 60 cases of cancer 46 would be correctly identified. A specificity of 95% would mean that out of

Table 10.2 Realistic frequencies for the outcomes of 10 000 screening mammograms.

	Cancer	Not cancer	Total
Positive mammogram	46	497	543
Negative mammogram	14	9443	9457
Total	60	9940	10 000

9940 disease-free cases, 9443 would be correctly identified as disease-free, leaving 497 false positives. It follows that a total of 543 cases would be identified as cancer: 497 disease-free cases plus 46 disease cases. If you had a positive mammogram, the likelihood of your having cancer is therefore 46/543 or around 0.08.

We can do the same calculation using Bayes' theorem. In the above data, the probability of a positive mammogram if cancer is present, $p(s|d)$, is 0.77. The prior probability of cancer, $p(d)$, is $6/1000 = 0.006$. The probability of a positive mammogram, $p(s)$, is $543/10\,000 = 0.054$.

By Bayes' theorem,

$$
\begin{aligned}
p(d|s) &= p(s|d) \times p(d)/p(s) \\
&= 0.77 \times 0.006/0.054 \\
&= 0.08.
\end{aligned}
$$

Reassuringly, it gives the same conclusion. Even if we allowed mammography to have a sensitivity of 90% and a specificity of 95%, a positive test result would only mean a 1 in 10 chance of having the disease. The odds would be even worse (or better, depending on your point of view) for a less common condition. It is difficult to make screening work as an intervention. You inevitably end up with high numbers of false positives. It is only worthwhile if early detection gives a substantial additional benefit and if the consequences of the false positives are not too severe (see Box 10.1).

An understanding of probabilities is therefore important in the interpretation of test results, it is equally important for making decisions about when a test should or should not be ordered. In the rest of this chapter we look at three different ways of using probabilities in decision-making: decision analysis, influence diagrams and Markov models.

Decision analysis

The following example is taken from a detailed and readable account of decision analysis, a book that I would recommend to readers who wish to take the subject further[3]. Before the discovery that cowpox could be used as a vaccination for smallpox, it was known that an inoculation of smallpox could protect against the disease. The problem was that the inoculation itself carried a risk of death. Benjamin Franklin wrote:

> In 1736 I lost one of my sons, a fine boy of 4 years old, by the smallpox taken in the common way. I bitterly regret that I had not given it to him by inoculation. This I mention for the sake of parents who omit that operation, on the supposition that they should never forgive themselves if a child died under it. My example shows that the regret may be the same either way and that therefore the safer should be chosen.

Box 10.1 Computer-aided detection in mammography

The lifetime risk of breast cancer is 1 in 9 for women in Britain and more than 40 000 British women are diagnosed with breast cancer each year[1]. The scale of the problem has led to the setting up of a national screening programme that invites all women aged between 50 and 64 for mammographic screening every 3 years. A mammogram is a planar X-ray of the compressed breast. All the signs used to identify potential cancers on mammograms can also appear, albeit sometimes in a slightly different form, as a result of non-malignant processes. Inevitably in screening, the vast majority, perhaps 99.4% of women, are disease-free[2]. The interpretation of screening mammograms is therefore a highly skilled and specialised task, which involves weighing up the risks of missing a possible cancer against the threat of overwhelming the programme with the unnecessary recall of healthy women.

The advent of digital mammography has led many researchers to consider whether computer algorithms could be devised that would automatically identify the signs of cancer on mammograms. Algorithms have been developed that can detect the most common signs of cancer[3]. These algorithms can be made extraordinarily sensitive. All of this might seem incredibly promising. There is, however, a catch. The sensitivity of the computer algorithms is only achieved at a considerable cost in terms of specificity and a screening test must not only be sensitive but also specific. It is all very well for a computer system to detect 98% of cancers, but if, in doing so, it erroneously suggests that 50% of the healthy population has cancer, it is not going to be acceptable as a screening test.

The idea behind computer-aided detection (CAD) is that these kinds of high sensitivity–low specificity algorithms can be given a role, if used to complement the skills of the human reader. Digital images (either acquired directly through a digital X-ray machine or by scanning conventional film X-rays) are analysed by the computer. The results are then used to create 'prompts' that indicate areas on the image that might be worth a second look. The films – analogue or digital – are then displayed in the usual way and viewed by the radiologist. The difference is that before recording a final assessment, he or she will consult the prompts, which can either be available on a paper sheet or displayed on a screen.

CAD systems for mammography have been available commercially since 1995. The idea has now been applied to other modalities. There seems to be a significant market for such systems, particularly in the USA. The evidence about the effectiveness of the tools is, however, less clear-cut than the commercial success might indicate. The impressive figures for the sensitivity of the algorithms claimed by the manufacturers have not been disputed[4]. What is less clear is how frequently radiologists

(*continued*)

Box 10.1 Computer-aided detection in mammography (*continued*)

alter their judgements on the basis of the information the prompts provide. There are, essentially, two forms of experiment that can be done to test this. One is to take a sample of films with known outcomes (normals and cancer cases) and have radiologists read them both with and without prompts and to test if the prompts make a difference. The other form of experiment, a prospective study, involves using a prompting system in the interpretation of real 'live' screening cases and comparing the radiologists' performance when prompted with some suitable benchmark. A number of groups have carried out both kinds of studies and the evidence is mixed. Some studies using films with known outcomes have shown a difference, others – including one large UK study – have not[5]. One prospective study has shown a 19% increase in the cancer detection rate[6]. Others have failed to show any increase[7].

The reasons for this variation are complex and, probably in part, to do with differences in experimental technique. It is likely, however, that one reason for the variation is that there is marked variation in the difficulty of cases – even studies with large numbers of cases will often involve only small numbers of cancers – and in the performance of radiologists. It is hard to avoid the conclusion that the overall impact of prompts is small relative to these other factors. But this is surprising. The prompts ought to have quite a dramatic effect. We know that many (perhaps as many as 25%) of detectable cancers are missed at screening[8]. We know that many (perhaps 90%) will be prompted. The problem is that radiologists repeatedly fail to recall cases with prompted cancers. At first glance this seems surprising; how can a radiologist not notice a cancer when the computer has placed a prompt over it? The answer is probably that the radiologist notices it but misinterprets the image and comes to the view that the woman need not be recalled. Part of the problem is the low specificity of the prompts. The prompts are like a burglar alarm that is always going off inappropriately. To extend the metaphor, the radiologist is like a dutiful security guard who always responds to the alarm, but who places a low value on the alarm in deciding how much time and attention to devote to the response.

This problem is just one example of a general problem in health informatics to do with how to make information available effectively. When is it appropriate to interrupt a clinician with an alert or some form of automatically generated reminder? At what point do people ignore alarms that occur repeatedly? How does the risk associated with failing to post an alert compare with the risk associated with devaluing the significance of the alert?

References

1. Cancer Research UK. *Specific Cancers: Breast Cancer.* http://www.cruk.org.uk/aboutcancer/specificcancers/breastcancer (accessed on 24 May 2004).
2. Patnick J (ed.) *Breast Screening Programme Annual Review 2001.* NHS Breast Screening Programme, England: Sheffield, 2001.
3. Warren Burhenne L J, Wood SA, D'Orsi CJ, Feig SA, Kopans DB, O'Shaughnessy KF, Sickles EA, Tabar L, Vyborny CJ, Castellino RA. Potential contribution of computer-aided detection to the sensitivity of screening mammography. *Radiology* 2000;215(2):554–562.
4. http://www.r2tech.com
5. Taylor P, Champness J, Given-Wilson R, Potts HWW, Johnson K. An evaluation of the impact of computer-based prompts on screen readers' interpretation of mammograms. *Br J Radiol* 2004;77:21–27.
6. Freer TW, Ulissey MJ. Screening mammography with computer-aided detection: prospective study of 12,860 patients in a community breast center. *Radiology* 2001;220:781–786.
7. Gur D, Sumkin JH, Rockette HE, Ganott M, Hakim C, Hardesty L, Poller WR, Shah R, Wallace L. Changes in breast cancer detection and mammography recall rates after the introduction of a computer-aided detection system. *JNCI* 2004;496:185–190.
8. Taylor P. Computer aids for detection and diagnosis in mammography. *Imaging* 2002;14:472–477.

But which way was the safer? In 1721 Zabdiel Boylston, faced with an epidemic of the disease, inoculated 286 Bostonians, of whom 6 died. In the larger population, of around 10 000, there were 5759 cases of the disease, of whom 885 died. If we use these numbers to calculate probabilities we can draw up the tree illustrated in Figure 10.1. The square represents a branching due to a decision we take. A circle represents a branching where chance comes into play. There is one decision, to inoculate or not, and there are three branches due to chance. To calculate which is the right decision we need to do three things:

1 associate each outcome with a value or utility;
2 calculate the probability of each outcome occurring; and
3 add up the 'expected utility' for each decision option, where expected utility is the utility of an outcome multiplied by its probability.

Let us assume that the utility of each branch that ends in life is 1 and the utility of each branch that ends in death is 0. The probabilities of the two branches that follow from inoculation are simply the probabilities of dying after inoculation (6/286) and of not dying (280/286). The probability of dying from smallpox is the probability of catching the disease (5759/10 000 = 0.58) times the probability of dying having caught it (85/5759 = 0.15) or $0.58 \times 0.15 = 0.09$. The probability of surviving smallpox is $0.58 \times 0.85 = 0.49$. The probability of escaping altogether is 0.42.

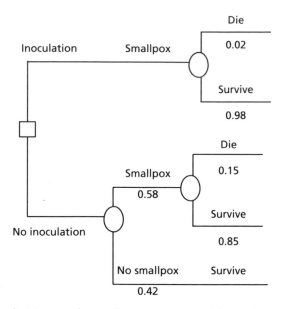

Figure 10.1 The decision tree for smallpox inoculation. Adapted from [3].

To sum the expected utilities of the two decision options, we take the expected utility of all the branches that end in death to be 0, and those of the others to be given by the probability. The total expected utility from inoculation is 0.98, from not inoculating is $0.42 + 0.49 = 0.91$. We can therefore see that inoculation is the safer course. Since the risk difference is 0.07 we would have to inoculate $1/0.07 = 14$ people in order to save a life. This way of presenting probabilities, the number of people treated for each person who benefits, is sometimes called the 'number needed to treat' and is often used as a measure of the effectiveness of an intervention.

The aim of decision analysis is to help work out for a particular decision what is the preferred selection from among a number of competing choices. It can be used to help patients work out what is the best course for them when faced with difficult choices about, for example, potentially risky treatments with uncertain outcomes. It is used by health providers to work out which interventions or public health programmes are worth funding. It can be used by health care professionals to determine when it is worth calling for additional investigations before starting treatment.

The justification for decision analysis is that, in certain situations, we find it difficult to make such decisions on the basis of a simple appraisal of the available facts, if, for example, there are different possible outcomes from each of the courses of action we might take, and these outcomes are associated both with differing likelihood and with consequences that we feel differently about.

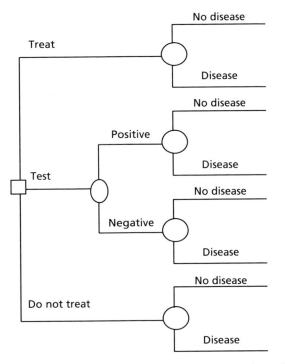

Figure 10.2 A decision tree for the decision to treat, not treat or investigate further.

Decision analysis and diagnostic tests

Consider a more complex example involving a decision about whether or not to order a test. The problem can be characterised as a choice between three courses of action: treat, do not treat or order a diagnostic test. The test may turn out positive or negative, correct or incorrect. Similarly both the treat and do not treat options have different outcomes depending on whether or not the patient has the disease. A simplified version of the resulting tree is presented in Figure 10.2.

I say simplified because I have not included branches to take into account the different possible outcomes of treating or not treating the disease. In most examples, some untreated diseased patients will recover and other patients will receive treatment but not respond, so we need a further level of branching to express the probabilities associated with these outcomes. There are other possibilities that we might want to take into account, there might be significant risks of side-effects associated with the treatment, and perhaps other risks associated with the test. We would need to have a measure of both the probability and the utility of the possible outcomes associated with these risks. For the sake of this example let us assume that all treated patients suffer some side-effects, that patients who receive the test suffer minor discomfort and that all patients with the disease recover if treated but only if treated. Let disease-free survival have a utility of 1, reduced to 0.9 by the side-effects of treatment with a further reduction of 0.01 for the test. Let the untreated disease lead to a reduced quality of life, having a utility of 0.5. Assume that 40% of the patient group have the disease and that the sensitivity and specificity of the test are both 90%.

The expected utility in the treat-them-all branch is then 0.9 per patient, since everyone survives but with the side-effects of treatment. In the treat-no-one-branch 60% end up with 100% utility but 40% have a utility of 0.5, giving a utility of 0.8 per patient. Consider the option in which patients are tested, in a sample of 100 patients, of the 60 healthy patients, 6 will end up as false positives – an outcome with a utility of 0.89, given the side-effects of both test and treatment. Of the 40 patients with the disease, 36 will be true positives; they too end up with a utility of 0.89. The 54 true negatives have a utility of 99, being tested but not treated, whereas the 4 false negatives are tested and not treated, so have a utility of 0.49. The expected utility of testing adds up to 0.92. It follows that testing before treatment is the rational course.

One can take a slightly more sophisticated approach to the problem and, taking into account some of the factors that we ignored above, determine a treatment threshold and a test threshold for a given test. These thresholds are used by clinicians to determine, on a patient-by-patient basis, whether it is worth ordering a test. If the clinicians' prior assessment of the likelihood of illness is above the treatment threshold, then it is not worth ordering the test because, given the probabilities and utilities for this case, there is sufficient concern to warrant treatment without the test. If the prior probability is below the test threshold, then it is not worth ordering the test, since even a positive test result will not raise the probability enough to indicate treatment.

Decision analysis can be used:
- to guide individuals in cases where their individual preferences combine with data about the probabilities of different outcomes;
- by health professionals to work out what level of confidence in a diagnosis is a sufficient basis for treatment;
- by policymakers to determine the appropriateness of a population-level intervention.

Broad as this range of applications is, the technique is limited in a number of ways. Clearly there are going to be situations where it is not possible to set out in advance exactly what all the options are. It is not a natural way to represent decisions where the choice is not a matter of what to do but of when to do it. Very often we do not know exactly what the probabilities of the different possible outcomes are. Most obviously, it is always, or almost always, difficult to associate a value with each of a set of possible outcomes. In the next section I consider some of the techniques that can be used to establish patients' utilities.

Utilities: measuring the desirability of outcomes

The aim of decision trees is to inform decision-making, specifically decision-making under uncertainty. The approach is a framework for calculating the expected utility of the outcomes that could follow from a particular choice, allowing the user to make a quantitative comparison of the available choices. The notion of expected utility, crucially, requires some measure of utility, of the desirability of the outcome.

The measurement of utility is not straightforward. It is easy to be sceptical about the idea that the desirability of a particular outcome, e.g. a state of health, could be quantified. It is as well to be honest about the difficulty: a measure of utility is not a measure of an outcome in terms of the patient's health or quality of life, but rather a measure of how he or she feels about the outcome. This is hugely complicated. Most of the cases where we feel the need to use something like decision analysis will be difficult problems involving many outcomes, each of which will have different attributes. A patient with prostate cancer, for example, has to weigh up the pros and cons associated with a procedure that could extend his life (but might not since prostate tumours are notoriously indolent) but which carries a significant risk of incontinence and of impotence.

There are a variety of techniques that can be used to determine how a patient feels about a possible outcome. The most obvious approach is to ask the patient to rate the outcome in question on some sort of scale, e.g. where 0 is death and 100 is perfect health. Another approach, known as the standard or reference gamble, asks the subject to judge what risk of immediate death they would accept in order to attain perfect health, in preference to their current or hypothesised state of health. Two other methods involve mapping utilities to units that are familiar from everyday life: time and money. Using 'time trade-offs' we ask patients to rate a state of health by saying how many years of life in that state they would give up in order to achieve perfect health. Finally a 'willingness to pay' analysis asks patients how much they would be willing to pay to achieve perfect health.

None of these methods is perfect. Each, to some extent, is measuring something different and produces somewhat different estimates of utility. Utilities obtained with the standard gamble are the highest – patients are very cautious when it comes to a risk of immediate death. Utilities elicited using rating scales are generally lower than the other methods. Such scales do not associate any real penalty with low ratings, and so patients are able to express negative feelings about a state of health without matching them against years of life lost or the risk of immediate death.

Eliciting an accurate numerical indication of utility is difficult. A further problem is that the numerical estimates may not work as they should when we try to use them mathematically. Let us assume for the moment that we have an accurate measure of utility. Let us call it quality-adjusted life year (QALY). For decision analysis to work a 50% chance of 10 QALYs should be equivalent to a 100% chance of 5 QALYs, just as a 50% chance of winning £10 should be equivalent to a 100% of having £5. But this implies that the person making the choice is neutral to the risk involved, whereas people have preferences for different levels of risk. These preferences vary even within individuals; most people are 'risk-averse' when it comes to major threats, as is shown by the fact that they take out expensive insurance against outcomes that are unlikely but that would have a significant impact, and yet many of the same people are 'risk-seeking' with small sums of money and prepared to hazard a pound or two on a lottery with an absurdly low chance of winning. A similar difficulty is that the mathematics requires that each additional QALY has an equal value. Most of us, however, worry less about years of life that are some way off. It is hard to persuade teenagers not to smoke using the argument that smoking might shave 7 years off the end of their lives. The same argument, however, would have considerable force for someone in the fifties or sixties. We can deal with this situation mathematically by 'discounting' future years.

The difficulties involved in eliciting and then making use of measurements of value are, as we have seen, considerable. The drive to have a solid, rational basis for important decisions is, however, such that a great deal of effort has gone into making the process as simple and robust as possible. There are health indexes or multi-attribute utility measures that allow a researcher to use a straightforward questionnaire to obtain information from a patient about his or her state of health and then to use data obtained from a reference population to derive a utility measure that reflects the preferences of the population in general. 'Off-the-shelf' utilities can be obtained from major studies to obtain an estimate of utility for a population.

An example: patient-based decision analysis in atrial fibrillation

Atrial fibrillation is a condition in which blood clotting can lead to stroke. Clinical trials have shown that warfarin, an anticoagulant, can significantly reduce the risk of stroke in these patients. However, others studies have shown that the condition is underdiagnosed and undertreated and it has been argued that this is because patients outside of clinical trials make different choices, being more tolerant of the risk of stroke and less tolerant of side-effects of treatment. Protheroe et al. carried out a trial in which patients and GPs used decision analysis to determine, on the basis of individual patient's utilities, whether or not to accept anticoagluation[4]. The decision tree is shown in Figure 10.3. The relevant probabilities were obtained from the literature and modified according to the patient's age and comorbidity. The time trade-off method was used to establish utilities. Of the 97 patients who participated, the decision analysis led 38 to decide against anticoagulation; of these 87% 'should' have been treated according to the agreed guidelines for this condition and 45% were being treated. Of the 59 who indicated,

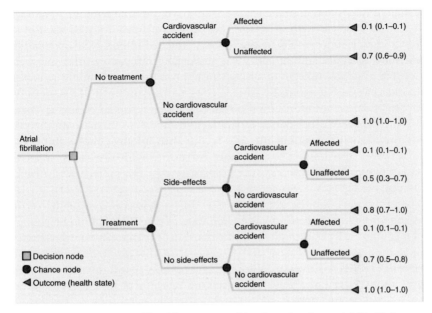

Figure 10.3 Decision tree of health states resulting from having atrial fibrillation, showing the mean and interquartile range for utility values associated with each state. From [4] with permission from the BMJ Publishing Group.

following decision analysis, that their preference was to be treated, 47% were not being treated. Of the 17 GP practices who were invited to participate only eight did and in these eight, decision analysis was carried out for only half the eligible patients, suggesting that the approach is not for everyone.

A systematic review of RCTs to assess the value of decision aids as an element in decision-making by patients found evidence that they improved knowledge, reduced decisional conflict and stimulated patients to be more active in decision-making, without increasing their anxiety[5]. There was, perhaps disappointingly, less evidence of an effect on satisfaction and an apparently variable effect on decisions.

Influence diagrams

Influence diagrams are an alternative to decision trees. Instead of representing a decision as a selection between alternatives, we model the impact of events on a desirable outcome or measure of utility. The diagrams show the chains of cause and effect and can be used, given the appropriate probabilities, to calculate the preferred course of action. They were developed, in part, through attempts to improve on the rather unsophisticated approach to Bayesian probabilities taken by de Dombal *et al.* in the AAPHelp system described in Chapter 1.

The use made of Bayes' theorem in AAPHelp is sometimes termed naive or idiot Bayes because the designers made a crucial simplifying assumption that the symptoms of abdominal pain are 'conditionally independent'. The starting point for the calculation was the set of prior probabilities for each of the seven diseases represented in the system: the likelihood that any patient, presenting with abdominal pain, was suffering from each of the seven diseases. The system worked by revising those seven prior probabilities given the information entered about the patient's signs and symptoms. If a patient was suffering from symptom A and the statistics showed this to be highly correlated with disease X, the revised probability would be an increase on the prior odds. Similarly if the patient was also recorded as suffering from symptom B, and this was also known to be highly correlated with disease X, a second revision would further increase the probability that this patient was suffering from disease X.

The problem is that the statistic used as the basis for calculating the second revision was a measure of how the likelihood of disease X should be changed given symptom B. This might sound right, but it is not. The correct statistic would be a measure of how the likelihood of disease X *in a patient with symptom A* is affected given symptom B. The point is that if the two symptoms were closely related, hearing about symptom B would be much less important in cases where the doctor had already observed symptom A. Getting the mathematics right, however, would involve collecting data not just about all the relevant symptoms but also about all possible combinations of relevant symptoms. The team behind AAPHelp knew that they could never contemplate this kind of data collection effort. Instead they collected enough data to revise the prior probabilities sequentially, on the assumption that any conditional dependence – to use the statistician's term – between the symptoms would not have a critical effect on the system's accuracy. An awareness of the vulnerability of the method to such conditional dependences must also have guided the selection of symptoms to include in the model.

Bayes nets

It is difficult to reason with large numbers of probabilities, unless we assume that they are independent. They cannot easily be combined. Probability is unlike logic in this respect. If we know the truth value of A and the truth value of B, then it is easy to determine the truth value of A and B. However, knowing the probability of A and the probability of B is not enough to determine the probability of A and B, unless we assume that their probabilities are independent. For this reason many successful applications of Bayes' theorem have made use of what are known as Bayes nets. These are graphical representations of the causal relationships in a domain that reveal the independence of different propositions. The diagrams consist of nodes linked by arrows. Consider the example in Figure 10.4a. Let us say that each node has two states: present and not present. To calculate the probability, for example, that a patient with a headache was suffering from stress and not a tumour we would need to calculate the probability $p(\text{not } A, B, C)$ which, by the fourth axiom of probability we know to be $p(C|\text{not } A, B) \times p(\text{not } A|B) \times p(B)$. The purpose of the diagram is to show that the probability of stress and the probability of tumour are independent, and therefore that $p(\text{not } A|B)$ simplifies to $p(\text{not } A)$. Similarly in Figure 10.4b the diagram shows that Kawasaki disease only influences the probability of chest pain because it can cause myocardial infarction. It follows that $p(C|B, A)$, in this example, can be simplified to $p(C|B)$. In Figure 10.4c we see that $p(B|A, C)$ simplifies to $p(B|A)$. The great thing about Bayes nets is that, however large and complicated the domain of interest, all we ever need to know is, for each state of each node, the probability of that state for each of the possible states of each of the nodes' parents: there may be many calculations but they are all local to a node and its parents, making both the data collection and the computation tractable.

Using Bayes nets

Consider the example in Figure 10.5. The example, which was first published by Speigelhalter, is taken from Krause and Clark's book, which provides a thorough introduction to the field[6,7]. The diagram can be used to calculate the probability of the various possible combinations of states for the different nodes. All we need to know is, for each state of each node, the probability of that state given each of the possible states of each of the nodes' parents. (By 'parent' I mean a node connected by an arrow pointing to the 'child' node.) The probability of, for example, 'severe headaches' $p(E)$ can be calculated as the sum of the probabilities for all the various combinations of nodes in which severe headaches are true:

$$p(E) = p(A, B, C, D, E) + p(\text{not } A, B, C, D, E) + p(A, \text{not } B, C, D, E)$$
$$+ p(A, B, \text{not } C, D, E) + p(A, B, C, \text{not } D, E)$$
$$+ p(\text{not } A, \text{not } B, C, D, E) + p(\text{not } A, B, \text{not } C, D, E)$$
$$+ p(\text{not } A, B, C, \text{not } D, E) + p(\text{not } A, \text{not } B, \text{not } C, D, E)$$
$$+ p(\text{not } A, \text{not } B, \text{not } C, \text{not } D, E)$$

Each of the ten probabilities in this sum can be calculated easily enough from the network. Take the first as an example. This can be calculated, using the fourth axiom of probability, as

$$p(A, B, C, D, E) = p(E|A, B, C, D) \times p(D|A, B, C)$$
$$\times p(C|A, B) \times p(B|A) \times p(A)$$

The network indicates that this simplifies to

$$p(A, B, C, D, E) = p(E|C) \times p(D|B, C) \times p(C|A) \times p(B|A) \times p(A)$$

Each of the five probabilities in this sum is given in the definition of the network. Given the prior probability of the parent node (metastatic cancer) and the various conditional probabilities, the prior probabilities of any possible combination of nodes and states can be calculated.

To make use of a Bayes network in a decision problem, we can use Bayes' theorem to update these prior probabilities when we obtain facts about a

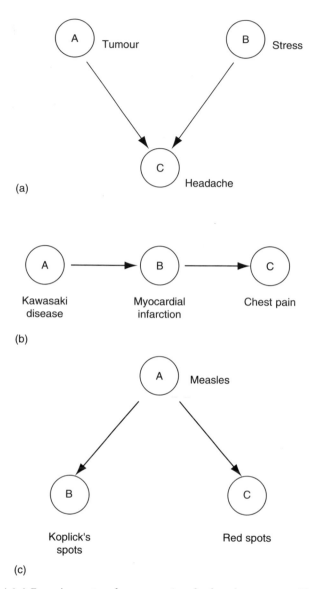

Figure 10.4 (a) A Bayesian network representing the fact that stress and brain tumour both cause headaches but that there is not a significant causal linkage between stress and brain tumours or any significant factor that can cause both stress and brain tumours. (b) A Bayesian network representing the fact that Kawasaki disease only increases the likelihood of chest pain because it increases the likelihood of myocardial infarction, a cause of chest pain. (c) A Bayesian network representing the fact that measles causes both Koplick's spots and red spots but that there is no other association between them. It follows that the probability of Koplick's spots in a patient known to have measles is not affected by the information that he or she has red spots: $p(B|A, C) = p(B|A)$. Adapted from [7].

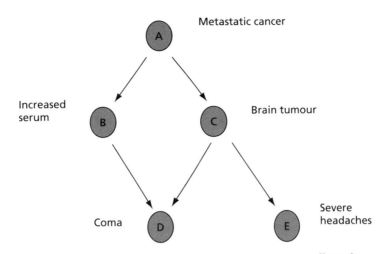

Figure 10.5 A Bayesian network showing how metastatic cancer affects the likelihood of both coma and severe headache. Adapted from [7].

particular patient. Imagine, for example, a patient who has a headache. We know the probability of headache given a brain tumour, $p(E|C)$; from the definition of the network, we can calculate as described above the prior probabilities $p(E)$ and $p(C)$. So we can now use Bayes' theorem to recalculate the probability of tumour, given the fact that the patient has a headache, p revised$(C|E) = p(E|C) \times p(C)/p(E)$. Propagating the values throughout the network involves a slightly more complex process, one beyond the scope of this book, but means that adding information about symptoms allows an accurate assessment of the probabilities of the different possible causes.

From Bayes nets to influence diagrams
A Bayesian network, as described above, does not explicitly represent a decision. It can be used to help make a decision but it does not explicitly represent the choices between different courses of actions or the utilities associated with different outcomes. We use the term 'influence diagram' to describe a Bayesian network that has been extended in this way. To turn the above diagram into an influence diagram we would have to add a node for an action, e.g. treatment of metastatic cancer, and links that indicated its impact on the likelihood of continued metastatic cancer. We would also have to augment the diagram with nodes for the outcomes of cancer and the utilities and costs associated with the outcomes and with the treatment. The model could then be used to determine the probabilities and utilities of the outcomes associated with the different courses of action.

Influence diagrams are an alternative formalism to decision trees. They have an advantage in that, being derived from Bayes nets, they are based on a model of cause and effect and so are a natural way to represent problems where the outcomes are determined by a set of competing possible causes. For many problems where a number of variables impact on a smaller set of outcomes, an influence diagram will be a more compact representation than a decision tree. The calculations involved are somewhat more complicated than those associated with decision trees, although the ready availability of software tools for building and using Bayes nets means that this is not the problem it might be. Readers with an interest in pursuing this approach are advised to download a freeware implementation and try out some simple problems[8].

Unfortunately there are some common problems in health care that are not easily represented using these kinds of diagrams. It is not easy to represent the passage of time in Bayes nets, so problems that involve estimating the risk of an event happening over a period of time are difficult. One technique that is often used for these kinds of problems is Markov modelling.

Markov models

A Markov process is one for which the future is determined entirely by the present. If we think of a process as a succession of time intervals (days, weeks, months, years), each of which may be in one of a number of states, then a Markov process is one for which the state at time $t + 1$ is determined only by the state at time t. This may seem a slightly arcane concept, but if we want to model a process, e.g. a disease, then if we assume that it is Markovian, we can model it very simply as a number of states (e.g. healthy, ill, dead) and the probabilities of the transitions between them. The Markov property means that the probability of a patient moving from one state to another (from healthy to ill, from ill to dead) is unaffected by the sequence of previous transitions. Consider the diagram in Figure 10.6. This shows a diagram used in an assessment of atrial fibrillation. Patients suffering from atrial fibrillation can be said to be in one of three states: well, recovering from stroke or dead. Patients with the condition who are being successfully managed have a roughly normal quality of life despite a significant risk of stroke. They may continue to be well but may suffer from a stroke, and may die. Patients who recover from a stroke will experience diminished quality of life and require different treatment. They are also at an increased risk of death. Death is, in the terminology of Markov modelling, an absorbing state, i.e. one from whose bourn no traveller returns. Building a Markov model is a matter of identifying the required states, the possible transitions between states and associating each transition with a probability or a range and distribution of probabilities.

In this example we give each transition a single probability, although it is quite possible to incorporate into Markov models more sophisticated analysis in which different patient subgroups are given distinct probabilities for certain transitions, and also to model probabilities that change over time (e.g. as patients get older). The probability is the likelihood that the given transition

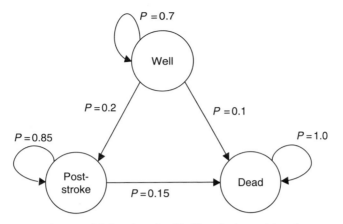

Figure 10.6 A Markov model showing the likelihood of transitions between three states: well, post-stroke and dead. Note the circular links that represent the probability of remaining in the same state. Death is an absorbing state; the probability of remaining in the state is therefore 1.0. Adapted from [3].

will occur within a defined time interval. One of the issues to consider in building a Markov model is what the time interval should be. Here it is taken to be 1 year. The choice of an appropriate interval will be determined in part by the clinical problem to be modelled, and in part by the nature of the available data.

Evaluating Markov models

To assess the impact of an intervention, one might want to use the Markov model to calculate the value of an appropriate outcome measure, for example, how long patients spend in each of the modelled states. There are three different ways in which a Markov Model can be used to obtain such a value. One can use matrix algebra to calculate from the transition probabilities what the expected time spent in each state will be for a population. One can use the model to calculate the proportions of a cohort who would move between states in a cycle and then calculate, after a number of cycles, what proportion of the cohort's total number of life years is spent in each state. One can also use the model to run what is called a Monte Carlo simulation in which the probabilities in the model are used in conjunction with a random number generator to simulate for individual patients, one at a time, their passage through the available states. The process is repeated for large numbers of patients (10 000) and the resulting data again used to calculate the proportion of time spent in each state. For most purposes it will also be necessary to associate some measure of utility for each state in order to determine what impact on the total utility of the population is obtained for a given change to the transition probabilities (see Table 10.3).

Table 10.3 The result of running the Markov model defined in Figure 10.6.

Cycle	Well	Post-stroke	Dead
0	10 000	0	0
1	7000	2000	1000
2	4900	3100	2000
3	3430	3615	2955
4	2401	3759	3840
5	1681	3675	4644
6	1176	3460	5364
7	824	3176	6000
8	576	2865	6559
9	404	2550	7046
10	282	2248	7469
...	...	...	...
63	0	0	10 000
Total	33 333	44 442	

Consider here how one might use the Markov model from Figure 10.6 to do a cohort simulation. Let us set the size of the cohort to be 10 000 and assume that all the patients start in the well state. The transition probabilities tell us that at the end of the first cycle there will be 7000 ($0.7 \times 10\,000$) well patients, 2000 ($0.2 \times 10\,000$) post-stroke patients and 1000 ($0.1 \times 10\,000$) dead patients. At the end of the second cycle, a further 1400 (0.2×7000) well patients have been moved in the post-stroke state, 700 (0.1×7000) well patients have died and 300 (0.15×2000) post-stroke patients have died. There are therefore now 4900 well patients, 3100 post-stroke patients and 2000 dead patients. After 10 years there are 282 well patients, 2248 post-stroke patients and 7469 dead patients. The last well patient succumbs after 28 years and the final post-stroke patient is only moved into the dead column after the 63rd cycle. The totals for the second and third columns show that 33 333 years are lived in the well state and 44 442 in the post-stroke state, respectively. It follows that the mean survival for a member of this cohort is $(33\,333 + 44\,442)/10\,000 = 7.8$.

One can use the model to see how a change in the transition probabilities would affect mean survival. Imagine a change in the treatment (say a change in the dose of anticoagulant) that reduced the risk of death from stroke, but increased the risk of stroke. We can alter the probabilities associated with the transitions so that the likelihood of staying well goes down to 0.675. The likelihood for going from well to dead goes down to 0.075 but that of going from well to post-stroke increases from 0.2 to 0.25. Under this regime, the total number of years lived in the well column sinks to 30 769, while the number of years lived in post-stroke rises to 51 280. Mean survival is 8.2. If that were the index on which the decision is to be made, it would seem that the new regime is a better one. A more sophisticated analysis would consider the differing utilities of years lived in the two columns and perhaps come to a different view.

Using Markov models

Canfell *et al.* (2004) used the Markov model shown in Figure 10.7 to examine the impact that changing the recommendations for cervical cancer screening would have on the lifetime incidence of the disease[9]. The model looks complicated compared to the simple example I gave earlier. The process starts with an uninfected state; next the model considers a state in which the patient has acquired cervical human papillomavirus infection. This can lead to the development of invasive cancer through a series of stages from microinvasive to frankly invasive cancer. The progression, however, is not straightforward; the disease can, at each stage, advance, persist or indeed regress. Patients may, at any stage, die from other causes. Patients in the later stages of the disease can be found at screening and, if treated, will return to an earlier stage: but not necessarily to uninfected. The authors carried out an extensive literature review in order to establish the transition probabilities required by the model. These include not just the transition probabilities associated with the model of the disease

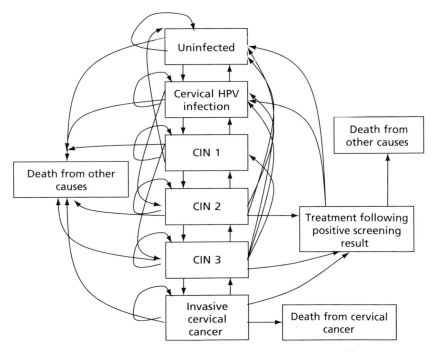

Figure 10.7 A Markov model showing states of cervical human papillomavirus (HPV) infection and cervical intraepithelial neoplasia (CIN) and invasive cervical cancer and the impact of screening on survival. From [9] with permission from Nature Publishing Group. © 2004 Cancer Research UK.

but also those that model the relevant parameters of the screening pro-gramme. Since the authors were interested in studying the impact of age-specific recommendations they needed to identify age-specific transition probabilities. In many cases the data that can be found in published papers will be in the form of progression or transmission rates and must be con-verted into a form that gives an annual transition probability. Running a number of simulations with the model, the authors were able to show that screening has little impact on women under 25 years of age, but that increasing the frequency of screening for women between 25 and 49 years of age from 3–5 years to 3 years has a significant impact.

Probability and decision-making

The history of attempts to improve clinical decision-making through the application of probability is now relatively long. I began this book with a discussion of the AAPHelp system, which dates from 1972. The impact of such systems, however, is still not great. A number of different explanations have been put forward for this, some of which were explored in Chapter 1. One argument was that probabilistic thinking is alien to clinicians, and that sys-tems dealing in probabilities cannot usefully be incorporated into clinical decision-making.

One proponent of this view has developed a rather different approach in which a decision is represented as a selection between alternatives but, instead of using mathematical calculations of expected utility to identify the preferred alternative, logical arguments for and against each of the alterna-tives are constructed and evaluated[10]. The method has a number of advan-tages: for example, arguments can be associated with weights that capture a notion of the strength of belief in the argument while allowing a degree of flexibility in how the weights are aggregated. Arguments can be evaluated, allowing 'meta-level' reasoning about the validity or suitability of arguments. The approach is particularly associated with reasoning about safety since it permits decisions to be evaluated according to a predefined safety policy. The approach has been incorporated in a variety of research projects notably in a system for the representation of clinical guidelines; this particular system is discussed in more detail in Chapter 13.

The important point to make here is that the crucial factor that determines the success of any attempt to model decision-making is not the method used to weight preferences. The most important thing is that the logical structure of the decision is right. If a decision tree, a Bayes net or a Markov model is not based on an accurate representation of the alternatives and the factors that effect preferences between alternatives, then the mathemat-ical precision of the method by which those preferences are compared is irrelevant.

References

1. Bayes T. An essay towards solving a problem in the doctrine of chances. *Phil Trans Royal Soc* 53:370–418, reprinted in Swinburne R, ed. *Bayes's Theorem*. Oxford: Oxford University Press, 2002.
2. Gigerenzer G. *Reckoning with Risk*. London: Penguin Books, 2003.
3. Hunink M, Glasziou P, Siegel J, *et al*. *Decision-Making in Health and Medicine*. Cambridge: Cambridge University Press, 2001.
4. Protheroe J, Fahey T, Montgomery AA, Peters TJ. The impact of patients' preferences on the treatment of atrial fibrillation: observational study of patient-based decision analysis. *BMJ* 2000;320(7246):1380–1384.
5. O'Connor AM, Rostom A, Fiset V, *et al*. Decision aids for patients facing health treatment or screening decisions: systematic review. *BMJ* 1999;319:731–734.
6. Spiegelhalter D. Probabilistic reasoning in predictive expert systems. In: Kanal LN, Lemmer JF, eds. *Uncertainty in Artificial Intelligence*. Amsterdam: North-Holland, 1986.
7. Krause P, Clark D. *Representing Uncertain Knowledge*. Oxford: Intellect Books, 1993.
8. Hugin Expert. *Hugin Expert Products and Services*. http://www.hugin.com/ (accessed 24 May 2005).
9. Canfell K, Barnabas R, Patnick J, Beral V. The predicted effect of changes in cervical screening practice in the UK: results from a modelling study. *Br J Cancer* 2004;91:530–536.
10. Fox J, Das S. *Safe and Sound*. Cambridge, MA: MIT Press, 2000.

CHAPTER 11

Probability and learning from data

In Chapter 3, three common ways in which patient data can be used to further medical knowledge were described: case studies, cohort studies and randomised controlled trials. I want here to look at the question of how we derive knowledge from experience in a more general, more abstract way and to introduce three sets of probabilistic techniques for analysing data and learning from it: statistical tests of hypotheses, machine learning and data mining. These are very broad fields and it might seem odd to deal with all of them in a single chapter; all, however, are based on the analysis of data-sets that includes some element of chance.

Falsificationism

The process by which a general principle is inferred from a set of examples is known as induction. If, for example, a sequence of patients who shared a set of symptoms all responded to a particular treatment, one might use a process of induction to infer that they were all suffering from the same disease. Philosophers regard induction as a problem because although this kind of inference is an essential element not just in scientific reasoning but also in everyday life, it is not guaranteed to lead to true conclusions in the way that deductive inference is. For example, there might be two different disease processes at work in these patients, and one might only respond to the treatment in certain circumstances. For a philosopher, this seems troubling; how is it, in the light of this uncertainty, that evidence from past experience can serve as a guide for action in the future?

One approach, much discussed in the philosophy of science, is to accept that we cannot ever know that a principle inferred from previous examples is true. All the laws of science are working hypotheses that we accept for the moment but that we have to be prepared to discard should we discover that the world is not quite as we thought. There is a useful asymmetry here: although no amount of positive evidence can ever definitively prove that a theory is true, a single negative result can be sufficient to show it to be false. This strategy, which is known as falsificationism, was first elucidated by Karl Popper, who wrote that 'the demand for scientific objectivity makes it inevitable that every scientific statement must remain tentative for ever'[1]. Science progresses not by proving new theories to be true but by discovering old ones to be false: 'Science never pursues the illusory aim of making its answers final or even probable. Its advance is rather towards an infinite yet attainable aim: that of ever discovering new, deeper, and more general problems and of subjecting our ever tentative answers to ever renewed and more rigorous tests.'

Although falsificationism is a good model for how scientists should proceed, it does not offer a very good model for living with scientific knowledge. Scientists believe that the MMR vaccine does not cause autism, and that the transmission masts for mobile phones do not cause brain tumours, but they know that they cannot be absolutely certain of their conclusions and hence find it difficult to couch them in terms that reassure the public. The account of falsification given here does not really do justice to Popper's thinking, and his work was not the last word on the subject, but the idea that science progresses by the falsification of theories has proved enormously influential. Later in this chapter, I will return to the idea of induction in the context of machine learning, but first I want to look at how, if falsificationism is accepted as an approach to scientific method, data can be used to subject our 'ever tentative answers' to 'ever renewed and more rigorous tests'.

Statistical hypothesis testing

In medicine, patient data are often analysed in order to test hypotheses. The data will generally be a sample from some population; for example, a trial of a treatment for hypertension might look at data from 50 patients, assuming that they are a representative sample of the larger population of patients with hypertension. Where the hypothesis involves comparing two samples (as in an RCT), the goal will often be to establish whether any difference between two samples is something other than the chance variation that might be expected between random samples. One way to consider this question is to calculate what is called a 'confidence interval' for the difference between the two sets of measurements.

Constructing a confidence interval

Consider a set of measurements, for example, of blood pressure. Such sets of measurements are often called distributions. We often want to summarise the information in a distribution. One useful summary statistic is the mean of the distribution. More information about the distribution can be obtained by calculating the average deviation of a measurement from the mean. This is called the standard deviation of the distribution. These two summary statistics, the mean and the standard deviation, tell us quite a lot about the set of measurements, about the distribution. Very often the distribution will take a characteristic form, a kind of bell-shaped curve with most measurements being pretty close to the mean, and relatively few being found further away, under the rim of the bell. This kind of bell-shaped distribution is called the 'normal' distribution. In a normal distribution, 95% of the observations will fall within a range of 1.96 standard deviations above or below the mean. I mention this specific fact because 95% is used, by convention, as a threshold in the calculation of confidence intervals.

If a sample from a population is large enough, the mean of the sample will be a good estimate of the mean of the population. In a smaller sample we might be less confident that its mean would be an accurate estimate of the population mean. The uncertainty associated with a mean estimated from a sample of a given size can be quantified by repeatedly sampling the population and observing how the mean varies from sample to sample. The means of the samples will be distributed around the true mean, the mean of the population. If the samples are large enough (e.g. greater than 100), the distribution of the sample means will be normal. It follows that 95% of the sample means will be within 1.96 standard deviations above or below the population mean. Note here that we are talking about the standard deviation of the distribution of the sample means, not the standard deviation of the measurement in the population. Luckily, the standard deviation of this sampling distribution is a simple function of the standard deviation of the measurement in the population:

$$\sigma/\sqrt{n}$$

where σ is the standard deviation of the measurement in the population and n is the size of the samples. We call this quantity – the standard deviation of the sampling distribution – the standard error (SE) of the estimated mean. Another equation can be found for the SE of the difference between the means of two sets of measurements:

$$\mathrm{SE}(x_1 - x_2) = (s_1^2/n_1 + s_2^2/n_2)$$

where s_1 is the standard deviation of the first set of n_1 measurements and s_2 that of the second set of n_2 measurements. A third equation gives the SE for a difference between two proportions:

$$\mathrm{SE}(p_1 - p_2) = \sqrt{\frac{p_1(1 - p_1)}{n_1} + \frac{p_2(1 - p_2)}{n_2}}$$

The SE can be used to construct what is called a confidence interval for a measurement. It can be said, with 95% confidence, that the true mean of the population will be within plus or minus $1.96 \times \mathrm{SE}$ of the measured mean. If mean blood pressures are calculated in two groups of patients, say from two arms of an RCT, it can be said, with 95% certainty, that the true difference between the means will be within a range that is plus or minus $1.96 \times \mathrm{SE}$ of the measured difference. If this range includes 0, then it cannot be said, with 95% certainty, that there is any difference between the means, suggesting that the study has not demonstrated any difference between the control and intervention group.

As Altman, on whose account the above presentation is based, writes, this procedure seems so straightforward that it may come as a surprise that most clinical studies are not analysed in this way but rather by the calculation of test statistics[2].

Calculating a test statistic

The traditional procedure for the statistical testing of hypotheses in medical research is as follows:

- Step 1 – specify a null hypothesis and an alternative hypothesis. The null hypothesis is generally that an effect is not observed, for example, that there is no difference between the control group and the intervention group in an RCT. The alternative hypothesis is the negation of the null hypothesis and is generally the hypothesis that the experimenter is testing.
- Step 2 – specify an acceptable threshold on the probability of drawing the wrong conclusion from the experiment. Conventionally a threshold is set only for the possibility of incorrectly rejecting the null hypothesis and it is generally set at 5% or 1%. These are sometimes called 'p values': the probability of observing the given value of the test statistic on the assumption that the null hypothesis is true. It is also common to talk about the significance level, or confidence level, so a p value of 5%, a 5% possibility of incorrectly rejecting the null hypothesis, would correspond to 95% confidence in the alternative hypothesis.
- Step 3 – choose a test statistic to be calculated from the data. The test statistic is the quantity that will be calculated from the experimental data and used to determine whether or not the null hypothesis is to be rejected.
- Step 4 – determine the critical value, also known as the significance point. This is a threshold on the test statistic. If test statistic computed for our experiment is greater than this threshold, the null hypothesis can be rejected with a certainty at least as great as that specified in Step 2.
- Step 5 – do the experiment, collect the data, calculate the test statistic, test against the threshold determined in Step 4 and draw the appropriate conclusion.

Step 4 dates from an era when the critical value was determined by consulting books of statistical tables, which listed the critical values for the standard test statistics at conventional significance levels: 95%, 99% or 99.9%. Now computers are used and the software will typically calculate the test statistic and its 'p value', making Steps 2 and 4 redundant.

Various forms of data and hypotheses

The choice of an appropriate test statistic depends on the nature of the data to be analysed, the form of the experiment and the hypothesis. Consider first the various forms that the data might take. Data vary in how they can be treated mathematically. Measurements of height or weight, for example, can perfectly sensibly be multiplied or divided. Such measurements are made on what is called a ratio scale. If the data consist of measurements on a scale that

Box 11.1 Statistical process control

It is easy to collect data. The difficult thing is to analyse them so that they can become a guide to action. We can collect data about, for example, the mortality rates of children following open-heart surgery in different hospitals. But what are we to do with this information? If we looked at the data there would be some variation, inevitably. How much variation should we expect? Most of the measurements will cluster around the mean, but a few will, inevitably, be scattered further away. How far away could they be before it should become a cause of concern?

Much of medical statistics is to do with testing for a hypothesised difference between two groups and involves studying how the data are distributed. The shape of the distribution will depend on the nature of the process being measured; for example, if the measure is of the number of discrete events that take place during a time interval of given length (e.g. patient deaths per annum), the sample will have a Poisson distribution. The number of independent measurements taking a value in a particular range (e.g. the height of patients in a particular group) will tend to have a Gaussian or normal distribution.

But what if we are not running a trial and we do not have a hypothesis that we wish to test? What if we are simply trying to analyse the variation to see what, if anything, needs to be done to improve quality or maintain patient safety? One approach, known as statistical process control (SPC), is to attempt to distinguish 'common cause' from 'special cause' variation. The idea is to measure the variation within a sample and identify cases where the variation seems sufficiently extreme to warrant attention. To test for 'special cause variation' we must first decide what proportion of the distribution counts as extreme, how far along either extremity to set the threshold so that a data point lying beyond the threshold is said to be 'special cause variation' and therefore worthy of investigation. We generally measure variation in units known as standard deviations. In SPC, the threshold on variation is conventionally set at three standard deviations from the mean. At this threshold, 0.27% of plotted data can be expected to fall in the extremities. Hence, a typical plot, which might contain 30 or so points, will very rarely contain a point in the extremity, unless it is there because the data item at that point is not part of the same distribution as the other items, i.e. it reflects some 'special cause variation'.

The basic analytical tool in SPC is a graphical device called the control chart. The technique is commonly used to look for fluctuations in measurements taken of a process at different points in time. The measurements are plotted, with the measured value on the y-axis and time point of the measurement on the *x*-axis. The quality of the process is assessed by looking for special cause variation. The task can be made easier by superimposing on the plot a grey line to indicate the mean and black lines at three standard deviations above and below the mean, these two thresholds are referred to in SPC as the upper and lower control limits.

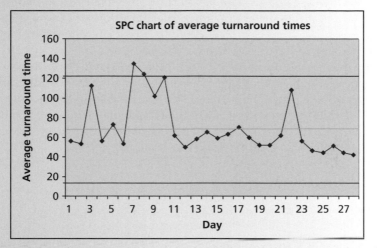

A control chart showing mean turnaround times for pathology tests over a 28-day period. The data show the spread of the points around a mean, drawn in grey. The dark horizontal lines indicate the upper and lower control lines. Two data points, days 7 and 8, are above the upper control limit and suggest special cause variation.

SPC was developed in the 1920s and first used to study processes in manufacturing. It has only relatively recently been used in health care[1]. It has been adopted with some enthusiasm by agencies such as the NHS Modernisation Agency, a body set up to identify and remove unnecessary delays preventing access to care. SPC has now been applied by a variety of agencies and teams with an interest in quality to a range of problems in health care, including, controversially, looking for GPs or GP practices with unusually high death rates.

British GP Harold Shipman was convicted of the murder of 15 of his elderly patients but is believed to have killed many more, perhaps as many as 215. It seems absolutely unbelievable that murder on such a scale could go undetected. But it turns out that normal variation could mask quite substantial 'excess mortality'. Frankel *et al.* considered the possibility that any practice in the top 0.5% of the Poisson distribution

(*continued*)

Box 11.1 Statistical process control (*continued*)

should be investigated[2]. With a list the size of Harold Shipman's (3600), an average of 40 deaths would be expected each year and the threshold for investigation would be 58. They conclude that this would allow an excess of 18 deaths per year above the average to pass as unremarkable. Clearly, however, the likelihood is that normal fluctuation of the natural death rate around a mean of 40 would fairly quickly mean that someone killing significant numbers would find themselves under investigation. Mohammed *et al.* argue that Shipman did stray outside SPC control limits derived from the district in which he worked[3]. Their analysis suggests 'special cause variation' in 1993, 1995, 1996, 1997 and 1998. The difficulty in using SPC as a kind of screening test, however, is that since there are 9000 practices in England, by a statistical inevitability, every year 45 would be in the top 0.5% of the Poisson distribution and would therefore come under investigation, creating what Frankel *et al.* refer to as a 'statistical cacophony of false positive suspicion'.

References

1. Hart M, Hart R. *Statistical Process Control for Health Care*. Pacific Grove, CA: Duxbury, 2002.
2. Frankel S, Sterne J, Smith GD. Mortality variations as a measure of general practitioner performance: implications of the Shipman case. *BMJ* 2000;320(7233):489.
3. Mohammed MA, Cheng KK, Rouse A, Marshall T. Bristol, Shipman, and clinical governance: Shewhart's forgotten lessons. *Lancet* 2001;357(9254): 463–467.

does not have a true zero, the differences between measurements can be compared but ratios cannot sensibly be computed. For example, if today the temperature is 4°C and yesterday it was only 2°C, we can say that it is hotter and indeed that the difference is 2°. We cannot, however, sensibly say that today is twice as hot as yesterday. This is because the 0 point on the temperature scale is not a true 0. Such scales are called interval scales. When users are asked to express their preferences by rating, for example a state of health, on a numerical scale, it makes sense to say that an outcome rated as 4.5 is better than one given a rating of 3. It would, however, be unsafe to assume that this difference is really the same as that between a state rated 0 and another rated 1.5. Such data are recorded on an ordinal scale, one that allows ranking but not statements about the distances between ranks. Other data might involve assigning patients, or whatever it is that is being studied, to a set of categories, where the categories are not ordered in any way: male and female or smoker and non-smoker.

Different test statistics are appropriate for different kinds of data. It is not just a matter of whether the data are collected on an interval or ratio scale but also of how they are distributed, for example, whether a normal distribution can be assumed. There are other issues too such as whether the data are repeated measurements on individuals or a comparison between two different groups of patients. As well as testing to see if there is a difference between two distributions, we sometimes want to test other kinds of hypotheses, for example, to determine if there is a correlation between two sets of measurements, or to determine – a similar but different notion – to what extent two sets of measurements agree. (Note: A statistical test of correlation is a test of the hypothesis that there is a relation between the measurements of two distinct properties: e.g. blood pressure and alcohol consumption; a measurement of agreement is a comparison of two attempts to measure the same properties. Researchers often test the statistical significance of a correlation, to determine the confidence with which it can be said that the detected association is not a random alignment of data points. It does not make sense to ask the same question about agreement, so although there is a statistical *measure* of agreement, there is not a statistical *test* of agreement. The extent to which the obtained agreement in a study is better than chance is calculated using a statistic called Kappa. It is not, however, easy to establish a significance point or a *p* value from this statistic.)

Test statistics

It would not be appropriate to provide a comprehensive survey of the variety of test statistics that are used in medical research. There are numerous excellent textbooks to which the interested reader can refer[2]. In the above account of how a confidence interval could be calculated, reference was made to the idea of a sampling distribution, which was said to take the form of a normal distribution for large sample sizes. Many test statistics are interpreted with reference to the statistic's distribution. Here I give a short summary of two, the *t* test, based on the *t* distribution and the Chi squared test, based on the Chi squared distribution. There are other tests that can be used in situations where the parameters of the sampling distribution are not known or cannot be estimated. These are often called non-parametric tests.

The *t* test

In describing the account of confidence intervals, I noted that for large samples from a population, the distribution of sample means forms a normal distribution about the population mean. For small samples, the distribution takes a slightly different form called the *t* distribution. The shape of the *t* distribution is determined by a single parameter, the number of 'degrees of freedom', roughly speaking the sample size of the study minus number of groups in the analysis. There are a number of statistical tests that use this distribution. Consider a clinical trial using interval or ratio data obtained from two independent samples (e.g. a control group and an intervention group) where the hypothesis is that there is a difference between the means; a form of the t test can be used, for which the test statistic is the difference between the two means divided by the SE of the difference between the two means. The obtained value of the test statistic is then tested against the distribution of t with $n - 2$ degrees of freedom where n is the sum of the sample sizes in the two samples, to determine the p value.

Chi squared test

Consider a different kind of experiment, one in which the data can usefully be summarised in a table. Consider, for example, a set of r categories that relate to social class and a set of c categories that relate to access to the Internet summarised in a table with r rows and c columns. Imagine that the null hypothesis is that there is no association between social class and Internet access. The appropriate test statistic for such an experiment would be the Chi squared statistic:

$$\chi^2 = \sum \frac{(O - E)^2}{E}$$

where O is the observed frequency in a cell, and E the expected frequency. The expected frequency of a cell in the ith row and jth column is estimated as the product of the total for row i and the total for column j, divided by the total for the table as a whole. The obtained value for the test statistic is then tested against the distribution of Chi squared to determine the probability that these data would be obtained if the null hypothesis were true, a probability that gives us a p value for the experiment. The Chi squared distribution has a very different shape to the normal distribution. If χ is normally distributed, χ^2 has a Chi squared distribution. If we have a set of N independent variables, each of which is normally distributed, the sum of the squares of each will be a Chi squared distribution with N degrees of freedom.

Correlation, regression and discriminant analysis

In the above example, the experiment involved testing for an association between two properties measured using categorical data. Where the experiment uses interval or ratio data, the degree of association between the categories can be tested using a measure of correlation. If both the variables are normally distributed, a plot of one against the other will result in a set of points, the scatter of which can be roughly described as an ellipse. The more the ellipse tends to a circle, the less likely it is that there is any association between the two variables, and the more it tends to a straight line, the more likely it is that there is an association. A measure of correlation, such as Pearson's correlation coefficient measures the degree of scatter around the underlying linear trend. A confidence interval and a p value can be calculated for the correlation coefficient allowing it to be used to test a hypothesis, for example, that there is an association between two quantities.

Where an association does exist between two quantities, it is possible, as described in Chapter 3, to use the association to predict a value for one quantity (the output value) given a value for the other (the input value). The statistical technique for this is called regression. Both correlation and regression involve identifying an underlying relationship between a set of points. A measure of correlation provides a test of the strength of association between two quantities, whereas regression provides a mathematical description of the association. This generally also provides a test of the strength of association; regression is therefore a more powerful technique.

The simplest form of regression is linear regression, which is used to identify the straight line that, in some sense, best captures the association between a set of points. A common approach is to find the straight line that minimises the average vertical distance of a point from the line. (Note: An alternative approach would be to use the perpendicular distances of each point from the line, but this would make the result dependent on the choice of scales for the two axes.) Once the regression line has been determined, it is easy to predict, for a given value of the input variable, an estimate of the output value. A statistical analysis of the scatter of points around the line will also allow the calculation of the confidence interval for that estimate.

A more complex variant of the technique is multiple regression, which attempts to describe the association between an output variable and a set of input variables. This can be performed using a stepwise approach in which each of the input variables is tested in turn to identify the one whose addition to the regression equation will most improve its capacity to 'explain' the data. A significance test is generally used to determine when it is no longer appropriate to keep adding input variables. A special form of multiple regression is non-linear regression, which is used to capture a non-linear association between the input and output variables. For example, if the association is best described by a quadratic curve, the equation of the regression line will take the form:

$$Y = a + bX + cX^2$$

This can be determined using a multiple regression techniques with X and X^2 as the input variables. The final variant of the technique is that mentioned in Chapter 3 that deals with categorical rather than continuous data. Instead of computing the output variable, a transformation of the output variable that has the appropriate mathematical form is computed.

Another statistical technique that involves finding a line through a set of data points is discriminant analysis. The aim here, however, is to find the line that best separates two classes of points.

Regression and discriminant analyses are complex statistical techniques, and it is not possible here to give more than a brief sketch of what they involve. They are, however, both extremely important to the theme of this book because they can be considered as learning algorithms. That is to say that they are used to analyse data from a set of example cases from which they derive a rule that can be applied to new cases. They induce a general principle from a set of examples. In the next section I consider a set of techniques, most developed from work in computer science rather than statistics, that allow computers to learn from experience.

Machine learning

The machine learning problem can be summarised in the following diagram, adapted from Vapnik[3] (Figure 11.1). There is some system that is under investigation. Data that are fed into the system are the input vectors (the term vector here just means a set of numbers), and data that are observed are the system's output vectors. There is some form of association between the two. The output might be a function of the input or there might only be a probabilistic association between the two, so that the output is a function of a conditional dependency of the input. Either way, there is some association between the two. The problem in machine learning is either (1) to identify the function that, in the system under investigation, generates the output, or (2) to identify a function that will, given the same inputs as the system, generate the same outputs, i.e. that will adequately simulate the behaviour of the system. We are here generally concerned with (2).

All this sounds very abstract. Consider a concrete example. We have a set of digital mammograms (breast X-rays) on which microcalcifications (traces of calcium salts) are visible. On some images, but only on some, the microcalcifications are caused by cancer. Some properties of the microcalcifications (branching shape, clustered distribution) are associated with a malignant interpretation; others are indicative of a benign cause. There is, however, no hard and fast rule to allow us to classify them. Might a computer be able to analyse the images, or measurements made from the images, and learn to classify calcifications correctly? The image data (or measurements made from

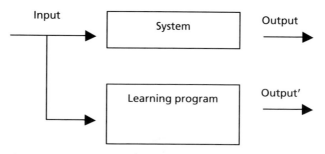

Figure 11.1 The machine learning problem.

the images) would be the input vectors. The output would be the classification (benign or malignant). This is an example of the simplest form of machine learning: pattern recognition. Imagine a two-dimensional plot of the data (with some measure of shape on one axis and a measure of clustering on the other); the output of the learning programme will be a function (not necessarily a straight line) that divides the benign from malignant cases.

If a program were trained to classify benign and malignant calcifications, that in itself might be useful. The resulting software, if sufficiently reliable, could be put to some clinical use. It might also be the case, depending on the approach we take to machine learning, that the rule used by the computer might tell us something about the microcalcifications that we did not already know. The rule learnt by the computer has been inferred inductively and it is as fallible as any other inductive inference. Any approach to inductive learning, however, is inevitably vulnerable to the possibility that the data used in the learning phase are not an adequate preparation for its subsequent use. If, in the above example, the images do not contain examples of all the possible forms of calcification, the rule induced from them will prove hopelessly inadequate. The following sections consider some approaches to machine learning, focusing particularly on classifiers.

Neural networks

The human brain is made up of cells called neurons. A neuron can be in one of two states: firing (transmitting impulses) or not firing. Neurons seem to function by aggregating impulses received from other neurons and, if the result passes some threshold, changing their state. Each neuron can be considered as having many inputs and a single output. It seems likely that when we learn, something is altered in the chemistry that controls the transmission of impulses between a pair of neurons so that the weights attached to certain inputs are altered, potentially changing the output.

Perceptrons

One approach to machine learning is to build computer systems that mimic this form of learning. For obvious reasons they are generally known as neural nets. The simplest form of neural net was devised by Minsky and Papert who coined the term perceptron[4]. A perceptron, as shown in Figure 11.2, has a set of inputs, each of which is assigned an inital weight. If the sum of the weighted inputs is greater than some threshold, the output is 1, otherwise it is 0. The perceptron is trained using a set of examples for which the correct classification is known. The process involves, for each example, calculating the sum of the weighted input values, seeing how the example is classified and, if it is not classified correctly, adjusting the weights. The process continues until all examples are classified correctly. Each of the possible combinations of weights is a hypothetical decision rule. The training is a search of the hypothesis space for a combination of weights that minimises a measure of

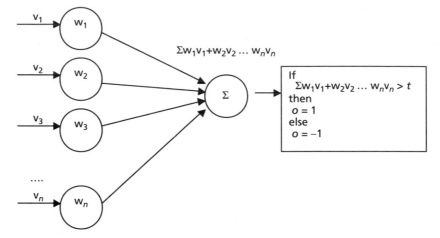

Figure 11.2 A single-layer perceptron.

'training error'. A common measure of the 'training error' associated with a set of weights $E(w)$ is

$$E(w) = 1/2 \quad \Sigma(t_d - o_d)^2$$

where o_d is the system's response to example d but t_d would be the correct, or target, response, the output. Assume for the moment that there is no thresholding step, and that the output of the perceptron is the sum of the weighted inputs. Perceptrons can be trained using an algorithm known as gradient descent. Imagine a system with just two inputs and hence just two weights w_0 and w_1. The hypothesis space is the w_0, w_1 plane. For each point in the plane one can compute a measure of E. These measurements form a surface. Although the shape of the surface will depend on the particular set of training examples, it will always be a paraboloid, having a unique minimum value. Gradient descent works by computing, for each training example, the gradient of E. At each step in the training the weights can then be modified so as to produce the steepest descent across the error surface, a descent that is guaranteed – in a parabola – to end at a global minimum, representing the optimum selection of weights.

Perceptrons can be trained to classify any linearly separable data-set. A set of example cases is linearly separable if the cases can be correctly classified by a single hyperplane. This is significant restriction. Figure 11.3 shows a two-dimensional data-set with just four examples but that is not linearly separable. (Note: A hyperplane is an n-dimensional surface. If the problem has only two inputs and can be presented in two dimensions, the data-set is linearly separable if the required classification can be made by drawing a straight line between the set of points. If there are three inputs, the data items are arranged in three dimensions and our linear separator will be a flat

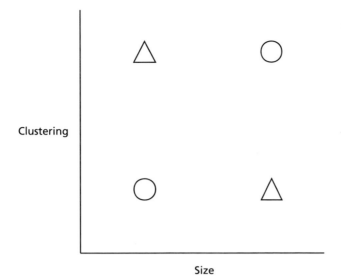

Figure 11.3 A simple data-set that is not linearly separable. Imagine that microcalcifications are detected on four mammograms (breast X-rays) and their size and degree of clustering are both measured. In two cases they are associated with cancer (shown as circles above) and in two cases they prove benign. If the data points fall as they do above, no linear classifier taking these cases as inputs would be able to learn a rule that would separate benign from malignant microcalcifications.

surface.) Multilayer perceptrons, neural nets that include at least one 'hidden layer' of neurons between the input and output nodes, can capture non-linear decision rules and, since they can have more than one output node, can capture multiway classifications.

Multilayer neural nets

Multilayer neural nets operate in an analogous way to perceptrons. There are two key differences. The output of each node is determined by a slight smoothing of the thresholding operation used in perceptrons, and, as shown in Figure 11.4, there is at least one 'hidden layer' between the input and output layers. The learning algorithm used is a modification of the gradient descent approach called back propagation. Each of the nodes in the input and the hidden layers is assigned an initial random weight. For each of the examples in the training set, the input values are used to generate output values that are propagated through the network. An error term is then calculated for each of the output and each of the hidden nodes. The error of a hidden unit is the weighted sum of the error terms for all the output nodes that it influences. The weight at each node in the network is then adjusted according to the learning rate (the step size used in calculating the gradient), the input value and the error in the output.

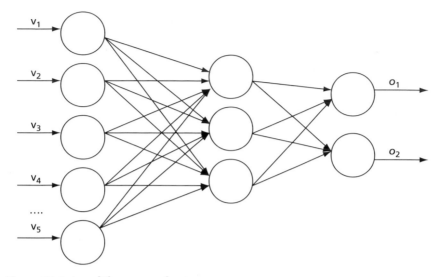

Figure 11.4 A multilayer neural net.

One of the problems with multilayer neural networks is that the error surface does not have the simple paraboloid shape it had for perceptrons. It can have many local minima, with the consequence that the gradient descent function is not guaranteed to find the optimal classification rule. Compared to other statistical approaches to machine learning neural networks have other disadvantages: the convergence of the gradient descent method is slow, and the learning rate has to be determined empirically. Advocates of other approaches to machine learning regard neural networks as poorly controlled; nevertheless, they are popular and have proved successful in a wide variety of applications[5].

Other approaches to pattern recognition

There are a number of other approaches that use machine learning to induce a decision rule. A common one is 'k nearest neighbours' in which a new example is classified on the basis of a vote taken by the k nearest neighbours in feature space, where k is chosen by the user. To go back to the micro-calcifications example, we must use data about the shape and clustering to classify images of microcalcifications as benign or malignant. If we have a set of microcalcifications with known classification and we want to classify a new image, we plot shape against clustering for all the images; if we choose a value of 5 for k, we identify the five points nearest to the new image, and if more than three of them are benign, we classify the new image as benign, otherwise we classify it as malignant.

Another approach to learning uses what are known as genetic algorithms. These work by analogy with evolution. The technique involves creating a set of potential solutions, e.g. hypothesised decision rules, and subjecting them to the processes involved in natural selection. There has to be a step in which 'genes' from different solutions are separated and recombined, as happens in mammalian reproduction. This step can also allow for small mutations to arise. There has also to be a step in which the 'fitness' of the various solutions is tested, to ensure that better approximations to the optimal solution are more likely to survive.

Two further approaches are worth mentioning since they build on ideas that were discussed in Chapter 10, Bayes nets and Markov models.

Learning with Bayes nets

In Chapter 10, I explained how to use Bayesian networks to model causal relationships in a domain, and showed how this approach made probabilistic calculations involving many different factors tractable. One of the problems with Bayesian networks is that very often not all the information required to build the model is available. A great deal of research has gone into developing techniques for learning Bayesian networks from a set of initial data. There are different aspects to this. The two main issues are: revising the conditional probabilities between nodes and revising the structure of the network, and adding or removing links between nodes.

Consider the first problem in the context of the Bayesian network in Figure 11.5[6]. The nodes are arranged in four layers representing the risk factors, diseases, actual symptoms and reported observations. Note the causal connections between nodes in the different layers. Before the network can be used to calculate probabilities, conditional probabilities have to be entered describing how the states of each of the nodes depend on those of each of the parent nodes. In Chapter 10, those probabilities were taken to be fixed. Here we consider that the initial data used to build the model are sampled from a population and we take the initial estimates of the conditional probabilities to be prior probabilities that are then updated as new data is analysed with the model. The priors are generally modelled not as point estimates but as distributions in which the mean of the distribution represents our best guess and the variance is a measure of the uncertainty. The data can then be used to give a revised or 'maximum a posteriori' estimate of the conditional probability. This works well if we can assume that we have complete data and that the model parameters are conditionally independent. Learning a new network structure is a less tractable problem since the number of possible models is an exponential function of the number of nodes. One approach is to limit the search to a manageable number of 'good' models.

Hidden Markov models

A Markov model, as described in Chapter 10, consists of a set of states and a matrix of probabilities for transitions between states. In a hidden Markov model there is another element: the output sequence[7]. This is drawn from a set of observable data items. There is also another matrix of probabilities

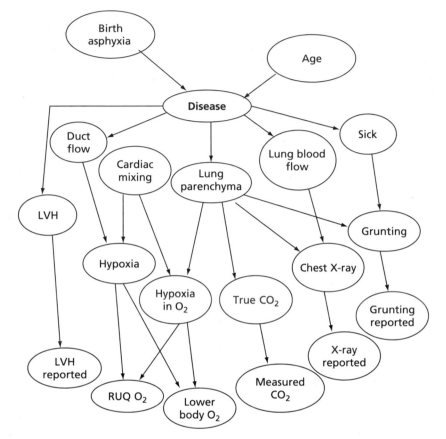

Figure 11.5 A four-layer Bayesian belief network in which risk factors (birth asphyxia and age) influence the likelihood of diseases, which in turn influence actual symptoms, which in turn influence reported symptoms. Adapted from [6].

that indicates how likely each of the observable data items is in each of the states. In a hidden Markov model, we observe the output sequence but not the state transitions. There are a variety of ways in which such models can be used. A common way is to attempt to predict the internal operation of some system of which we have partial knowledge. One algorithm, the Viterbi algorithm, allows the user to infer which of the possible sequences of states is most likely given an observed output sequence and prior knowledge of both the matrices of probabilities in the model. Another, the Baum–Welch algorithm, is used to infer, from a given output sequence, the most likely probabilities.

Issues in machine learning
This chapter provides only the skimpiest of introductions to a difficult and rapidly changing field. From the perspective of a student in health informatics

the principal lesson is that there is a wide variety of computational techniques by which new knowledge can be inferred from the analysis of data. It is worth pointing out some of the common themes that link these approaches. The idea, introduced in the discussion of perceptrons, that a decision rule can be considered as a surface in a feature space is a completely general one. Many of the methods considered can be viewed as attempts to search a hypothesis space that consists of all the possible decision rules, with the aim of minimising some measure of learning error. They are attempts to find an optimal solution to a problem with potentially many solutions (such problems are sometimes called ill-posed problems).

One of the difficulties in machine learning is that, if the search for a solution is unconstrained, the identified decision rule will 'overfit' the training data. If there is no limit on the complexity of the permitted decision surface, it will be too precisely moulded around the data points in the training set, which will lead to unpredictable consequences when it is tested against new data. In jargon of the field, it will fail to generalise. One approach to this is to apply some form of Ockham's Razor. This is a principle, traditionally attributed to a fourteenth-century English monk, William of Ockham, who wrote: 'Pluralitas non est ponenda sine necessitate', which translates into English as 'Plurality should not be posited without necessity'[8]. For our purposes, the idea is that there has to be some additional cost associated with increasing the complexity of the decision rule.

One of the most exciting recent developments in machine learning is an approach that incorporates a measure of the richness or flexibility of a decision rule. The measure is known as the capacity of the rule or, more technically, as its Vapnik–Chervonenkis dimension and it is used in support vector machines[9].

Support vector machines

Single-layer perceptrons can learn a linear decision rule: they can only separate points that lie on either side of a hyperplane. Support vector machines are a more refined form of linear classifiers that manage to avoid some of the problems associated with neural nets while finessing the limitation that the decision rule be a hyperplane. Much of the mathematics behind the method is beyond the scope of this book but a few points are worth making.

The first is that the basic idea in support vector machines is to identify the hyperplane that maximises the margin between the two sets to be classified. The margin is defined as the distance between the hyperplane and the points lying closest to it on either side. These points are referred to as the support vectors for the hyperplane. The other points in the training set play no part in the constraint and are irrelevant to the classification task. The choice of the maximum margin hyperplane as a classifier is motivated by a result from statistical learning theory, which identifies a lower bound on the likelihood that a decision rule learnt from these examples will fail to generalise to future examples[10].

The technique used in support vector machines to generalise from linear to non-linear decision rules is known as the kernel trick. The idea is to map from the original feature space into a higher-dimensional feature space. This increases the likelihood that a hyperplane will be found that can separate the examples in the data-set. Imagine a two-dimensional data-set that is not linearly separable, think of the points as if printed on a page. Imagine pulling the points off the page, as if they were connected to it by different lengths of elastic. The points are now scattered across a third dimension; perhaps a separating plane might be found that takes advantage of this extra scattering. The kernel trick does not guarantee that all the examples will be classified correctly; the aim in support vector machines is to find the optimal classifier but does not guarantee a perfect one. The extra dimensionality makes the required computations more costly but the cost can be contained if the mapping is well chosen.

Support vector machines are a relatively recent arrival, at least in terms of the application to machine learning problems, but they have proved extremely powerful and are likely to be used more and more frequently in applications involving learning from large and complex data-sets.

Data mining

The use of medical data in experiments, in tests of predefined hypotheses, is completely routine for researchers across all the various clinical specialities and indeed the life sciences. Yet only a tiny proportion of patients are ever enrolled in clinical trials. What might be learnt from data about other patients who are not recruited into such experiments, from an analysis of the data that the NHS collects routinely as part of the process of caring for its patients? When a researcher gets access to a large data-set, there is always a temptation to run a variety of statistical tests of different kinds and 'see what comes up'. The probabilistic nature of such tests means that if you run enough of them, eventually something will probably come up and when it does it may look like a pretty striking result, even though it is just a statistical artefact. A very different approach is to attempt to induce new knowledge from the data. This approach is called 'data mining' or knowledge discovery in databases.

Data mining is a similar but slightly different notion to machine learning. Data mining is a specific application area in which a variety of algorithms are applied, some but not all of which are drawn from machine learning. The issues in data mining are often a little different from those in typical machine learning applications, for example, the data-sets tend to be larger, and also somewhat messier; data mining is an applied field and therefore has to deal with the problems of real-life data-sets with incomplete or noisy data.

In addition to Bayesian classifiers, neural networks and support vector machines, statistical techniques for testing describing association are used. Data mining also makes use of other techniques, for example, for identifying clusters in data. One common approach is the k-means classifier, which groups a data-set into a number of clusters (usually a predefined number). The algorithm, which is yet another optimisation algorithm, seeks the minimum value for a cost function based on the mean distance between each data point and the centroid of the cluster to which it belongs. A common variant of the technique uses a fuzzy membership function to allow data points to belong to more than one cluster.

Data mining in pharmacovigilance

A major new clinical application area for data mining is pharmacovigilance. Adverse drug events are estimated to account for 5% of hospital admissions, 28% of emergency department visits and 5% of hospital deaths. Although the regulatory environment requires that new drugs undergo rigorous trials before they can be brought to market, post-marketing surveillance of drugs is crucial for the detection of harmful effects, which are only revealed after prolonged use, or when taken by patients in particular risk groups. The reporting mechanisms for adverse drug events have led to the creation of a variety of databases that can be used for data mining. These databases include spontaneous reporting databases, such as the UK Yellow Card scheme, monitoring schemes that collect high-quality data for select groups of patients exposed to new drugs, large linked administrative databases and electronic medical records[11].

A retrospective study by the US regulatory authority, the Food and Drug Administration (FDA), suggested that a Bayesian statistical analysis of their adverse drug event reporting database would have identified 20 out of 30 known classes of adverse drug events 1–5 years before their detection by existing methods. Hauben and Reich compared the FDA's Bayesian approach with another test of disproportionality, the proportional reporting ratio (PRR); they analysed data from the FDA to look for associations with pancreatitis and report that PRR identified 15 out of 16 previously recorded associations[12]. Interestingly, however, they note that the importance of sound clinical, pharmacological and epidemiological judgement is not diminished by the advent of these techniques, and that they are not yet at a point where they can be used in isolation. Over-reliance on data mining may be hazardous, since signal scores based on small numbers of events may be missed; also alerts may be generated that would readily be dismissed by a clinical review of the relevant cases.

Conclusion

This chapter provides a very brief introduction to a variety of approaches that can be used to derive new knowledge from patient data. This includes the broad and complex field of medical statistics and the more recent, and rapidly changing, fields of machine learning and data mining.

These techniques, especially the newer techniques of data mining and machine learning, are being used to great effect by bioinformaticians, uncovering some of the secrets hidden in the vast amounts of data generated by experiments in molecular biology. Machine learning and data mining techniques are also being used to analyse clinical data. A recent review of Bayesian networks identified applications in diagnosis, prognosis and treatment selection[13]. Examples of other applications include training Bayesian networks to identify patients having a low pre-test probability of venous thromboembolism, support vector machines for analysing statistical differences in anatomical shape and using neural networks in the derivation of staging criteria for cancer[14,15,16].

As the developments discussed in earlier chapters – controlled clinical terminologies, the use of ontologies and well-defined standards – progress, they will improve the quality and availability of data, which in turn will enhance and extend the scope for applying machine learning and data mining. These techniques will help identify new hypotheses from large data-sets and allow software to be designed for tasks that cannot be completely specified. They should not be overused, however. Better hypotheses will often be generated from a thoughtful inspection of data by an expert. Software based on a sound understanding of the relevant domain may well outperform classifiers trained in using machine learning techniques. The arguments are similar to those rehearsed at the end of Chapter 10. Machine learning approaches can extract information that a human being would never be able to detect in the data, but they can be led astray. It is often possible to get a 'quick win' by applying a neural network classifier to a problem, but it is better in the long run to tackle it by trying to understand the real underlying differences that should be used to classify the data.

References

1. Popper K. *The Logic of Scientific Discovery*. London: Hutchinson, 1959.
2. Altman D. *Practical Statistics for Medical Research*. London: Chapman & Hall, 1991.
3. Vapnik V. *Statistical Learning Theory*. New York: John Wiley, 1998.
4. Minsky M, Papert S. *Perceptrons*. Cambridge, MA: MIT Press, 1969.
5. Mitchell D. *Machine Learning*. New York: McGraw-Hill, 1997.
6. Krause P, Clark D. *Representing Uncertain Knowledge*. Oxford: Intellect Books, 1993.
7. Lesk AM. *Introduction to Bioinformatics*. Oxford: Oxford University Press, 2002.
8. Cristiani N, Shawe-Taylor J. *An Introduction to Support Vector Machines*. Cambridge: Cambridge University Press, 2000.
9. Hearst M. Support vector machines. *IEEE Intell Sys* 1998;13:18–21.
10. Wilson AM, Thabane L, Holbrook A. Application of data mining techniques in pharmacovigilance. *Br J Clin Pharmacol* 2004;57(2):127–134.
11. Hauben M, Reich L. Drug-induced pancreatitis: lessons in data mining. *Br J Clin Pharmacol* 2004;58(5):560–562.
12. Lucas PJ, van der Gaag LC, Abu-Hanna A. Bayesian networks in biomedicine and health-care. *Artif Intell Med* 2004;30(3):201–214.

13. Kline JA, Novobilski AJ, Kabrhel C, Richman PB, Courtney DM. Derivation and validation of a Bayesian network to predict pretest probability of venous thromboembolism. *Ann Emerg Med* 2005;45(3):282–290.

14. Golland P, Grimson WE, Shenton ME, Kikinis R. Detection and analysis of statistical differences in anatomical shape. *Med Image Anal* 2005;9(1):69–86.

15. Kates R, Schmitt M, Harbeck N. Advanced statistical methods for the definition of new staging models. *Recent Results Cancer Res* 2003;162:101–113.

Part 3
Achieving Change

CHAPTER 12
Information technology and organisational transformation

In 2001 the US Institute of Medicine (IOM) produced a report on the quality of health care in the USA[1]. Its authors concluded that between the quality of health care the USA had and that which it could and should have lay not a gap but a chasm. Four factors were said to have created this situation: the lag between progress in medical research and change in medical practice, that the system was chiefly organised for the delivery of acute care when the bulk of the demand was for the management of chronic conditions, inadequate use of IT and, finally, payment schemes that provided little or no incentive to improve quality. Since the report said the system was comprehensively broken and, further, that this was so in part because insufficient attention had been paid to IT, an argument might be made that a radical restructuring was required and that it should give IT a central role.

By the end of the 1980s, IT had dramatically altered the context within which many businesses were operating, with the result that IT was, when the IOM report came out, at the heart of thinking about business strategy and organisational transformation. Instead of using IT to make incremental improvements in existing ways of doing things, senior managers in corporations and businesses were encouraged to see the potential for transformational change. Writers on IT strategy argued that, instead of commissioning a new IT system to support the organisation, so that the latter served as a constraint on the former, it was better to redesign the business in order to fully exploit the capabilities of the available IT, so that the IT determined the shape of the organisation, not vice versa[2].

Businesses exist within networks of suppliers, buyers and intermediaries. Some of the opportunities for organisational transformation, therefore, will lie not within the boundaries of an organisation but in the surrounding network. Companies have traditionally exploited such opportunities through processes of vertical or horizontal integration. A vertically integrated company is one that combines business units at all stages of the process of production, for example, a media company that owns film studios, production facilities, distributors and cinemas or video outlets. A horizontally integrated company is one that increases its effectiveness by fulfilling the same function in different markets: e.g. a retailer that sells food and furniture as well as clothes. Networking IT systems makes it possible for businesses to achieve a level of functional integration while remaining distinct entities. One approach is to develop close relationships with partner organisations; another is to develop a standard IT infrastructure across all participants. These kinds of integration can take place at a variety of levels: automation of transactions, sharing of data across organisational boundaries, integration of processes and the sharing of specialised skills and knowledge.

The different forms of IT-induced transformation discussed above could be applied to health care at the start of the twenty-first century. There is substantial scope for the redesign of business processes within organisations and for a rethinking of the way in which networks of different organisations collaborate in the delivery of care. Many of the transactions that take place between health care organisations are now automated. For example, the results of tests carried out in hospital pathology labs are automatically downloaded to GP surgeries. The proposed electronic health care records will allow patient data to be shared between primary and secondary care organisations. Electronic booking, being implemented in the NHS at the time of writing, is a good example of the integration of business processes across organisational boundaries. Many of the initiatives described in the preceding chapters – SNOMED CT, openEHR, HL7, DICOM – can be seen as laying the foundations for levels of integration that will make possible different ways of organising the delivery of health care.

There ought, therefore, to be considerable potential for IT to drive the transformation of health care organisations. However, the literature on ways of achieving organisational change in the public sector suggests that radical revolutionary change is incompatible with the culture and traditions of health care organisations, such as those that make up the NHS. McNulty and Ferlie made an influential contribution to that literature with a detailed account of attempts to apply 'business process reengineering' in the NHS[3].

Business process reengineering in the NHS

These ideas about IT-induced organisational transformation formed a prominent part of a larger movement towards advocating the 'fundamental rethinking and radical redesign of business processes to achieve dramatic improvements in critical contemporary measures of performance such as cost, quality, service and speed'. A series of publications in the 1990s advocated the abolition of traditional departmental boundaries and a reorganisation around core business processes. The approach became known as 'business process reengineering' and was first applied in the US manufacturing sector but was rapidly adopted by managers in Europe and in the public sector. It is generally understood to include the following elements:
- a fresh start, radical holistic change that disregards existing ways of working;
- a top-down approach, relying heavily on individual leadership;
- a structure of teams and committees dedicated to reengineering;
- a focus on a small number of essential processes through which the work of the organisation is carried out.

These ideas arrived in the UK at a time when a new management culture was taking root in public sector organisations, such as the NHS. Public sector organisations were becoming more autonomous and managers were encouraged to become more entrepreneurial. A level of competition was introduced, with organisations such as NHS Trusts operating more like commercial businesses, and greater use was made of efficiency targets to achieve improvements in productivity. One trust, Leicester Royal Infirmary (LRI), having been involved in a quality improvement initiative through which services in neurology and hearing were successfully redesigned to reduced waiting times became, in 1994, a national pilot site for 'reengineering'.

McNulty and Ferlie present six case studies of attempts to apply reengineering at LRI: patients attending A&E with minor injuries, patients admitted with fractured neck of femur, elective surgery within gynaecology, outpatient services in gynaecology, elective surgery in ENT and outpatient services in gastroenterology. To get a flavour of the kind of work that was carried out and the degree of success achieved, consider two initiatives from the first case study:

> *Nurse-ordered X-rays.* Data collected by the reengineering team revealed that the biggest delay for patients attending A&E with minor injuries was waiting for a doctor to order an X-ray. Of all 'walking wounded' patients 40% required an X-ray and 80% of those were for minor injuries below the knee or elbow. The team therefore proposed that, for certain patients, X-rays be ordered by nurses of appropriate grades. This would reduce the initial wait and reduce the number of consultations medical staff had to perform.

> *Nurses carrying out simple treatments.* It was accepted practice that all A&E patients were seen by a doctor. The reengineers argued that 20% of patients could be treated by the triage nurse without getting into the queue.

These initiatives were slow to take off. The protocols intended to guide the ordering of X-rays took time to develop. It took 2 years to train even 75% of the nurses so that they were able to order X-rays and carry out simple treatments. After 2 years it was found that 56% of 'walking wounded' patients were having X-rays and nurses were ordering 78% of them; however, only 7.8% of patients were receiving simple treatments at triage. None of the performance targets was met and there was no evidence that waiting times were improved. It turned out that the A&E department was a difficult environment in which to achieve change. The department had a problem recruiting and retaining nursing staff, space was limited and the staff were not receptive to ideas for change. McNulty and Ferlie include many telling quotes from interviews with staff who clearly felt that the reengineers did not have an adequate understanding or experience of A&E work.

Some of the other initiatives were more successful, but the broad picture that emerges is, however, that rapid organisational change is hard to achieve. One of the interesting conclusions of the work is that although business process reengineering encourages managers to start afresh and disregard existing ways of working, much of what was done was determined by the existing organisational structures. The new 'process-based thinking' did not break down the traditional structure of directorates and clinical services.

McNulty and Ferlie list five further categories of factors that they argue explain the variation in impact of the various process reengineering initiatives. These deal with the organisation and management of the programme, the presence of a receptive context for change, the scope and complexity of the patient processes, the approach to change and the availability of resources. A clear overall conclusion, however, would be that top-down, externally imposed, radical change is unlikely to succeed in organisations like NHS Trusts.

Organisational change

The history of health informatics, as we have seen, includes many examples of promising innovations that have failed to have the anticipated impact. One possible cause is that the technology requires some kind of organisational transformation before the benefits can be achieved and that this kind of radical change is hard to effect in health care, for reasons that are to do with the kinds of organisation through which health care is delivered. What, then, can be achieved?

The topic of 'organisational change' has attracted a great deal of attention in recent decades, and a number of theories and approaches have been proposed. The literature in this area is difficult to review. Inevitably the interventions being studied are complex and many competing explanations could be offered for the success or failure of any 'change project'. It would be hard to conduct an RCT to establish whether one approach (e.g. business process reengineering) is better than any other. Iles and Sutherland present a useful summary, for health care managers and researchers, of approaches to organisational change with a review of the relevant literature[4].

They identify a large number of theories and frameworks, which they review under four headings:

- How can we understand complexity, interdependence and fragmentation?
- Why do we need change?
- Who and what can change?
- How can we make change happen?

Among the approaches to understanding complexity identified by Iles and Sutherland, there are a number that attempt to model processes. Only one approach is listed under the heading 'Why do we need change?', and that is the well-known technique of SWOT analysis, by which an organisation examines its Strengths, Weaknesses, Opportunities and Threats in an attempt to identify a mismatch between what it is doing and what it ought to be doing. Business process reengineering is discussed under the heading 'Who and what can change' as are a number of similar approaches to achieving 'organisation-level' change and also approaches to group- and individual-level change. There are four approaches that specifically address the question of 'how can we make change happen?': organisational development, organisational learning, action research and project management.

Organisational development

Organisational development is defined as 'a set of behavioural science–based theories, values, strategies and techniques aimed at the planned change of organisational work setting for the purpose of enhancing individual development and improving organisational performance through the alteration of organisational members' on-the-job behaviours'. Given the broad scope of the definition, it can be seen as an umbrella term for a wide variety of approaches. For example, improvement in the performance of an organisation can be achieved by improving the performance of the individuals that make up the organisation, but this may be achieved through a variety of changes, many of which alter the organisational setting: changing the organising arrangements, goals strategies or procedures, changing social factors such as the management style or social networks, changing the physical setting or the technology or work practices.

The practitioners of organisational development help their clients manage change in a variety of ways: assessing the need for change, designing the plan for change, helping others adapt to change and dealing with resistance to change. Iles and Sutherland cite several reviews that suggest that organisational development has, on the whole, proved effective as an approach to producing positive change.

Organisational learning

Organisations can transform themselves by using knowledge to change and improve. The process of learning can be adaptive, or single-loop learning, in which incremental change is carried out to narrow the gap between goals and outcomes. The proponents of organisational learning argue that this single-loop learning can be dysfunctional since it reinforces the assumptions underlying the status quo. Second loop, or generative learning, which challenges the conditions within which single-loop learning operates is advocated as a way of achieving transformational change. A third level of learning, learning how to learn, is directed at the learning process itself.

Iles and Sutherland identify little evidence of the impact of organisational learning in practice but note that the approach is becoming more popular with many organisations attempting to follow a model set out for learning organisations, developing structures that encourage innovation.

Action research

The concept of action research dates from the 1940s. The approach is defined in opposition to traditional empirical research in which the researcher attempts to maintain an objective stance and not to intervene in the situation being studied. In contrast, the action researcher engages with the situation and seeks to be involved in decisions about how to remedy problems. Action research, therefore, involves collecting data about a situation or a system, identifying a problem, taking action to alter the situation and collecting new data to assess the impact of the action. An important aspect of the approach is that the members or staff of the organisation should be active participants in the research and in the action; that they should be involved in articulating the problem, planning the intervention and taking it forward. The approach has been widely applied and the literature reviewed by Iles and Sutherland includes a number of examples of its successful application.

Project management

There is a well-established definition of a project, involving a number of features. A project is generally understood to have a specified goal, it is something that is carried out once and it has limited duration. A project normally has a manager who has a set of resources: money, people and materials with which to achieve the project goal. Not all change interventions meet this definition, not all change is achieved through the completion of well-defined projects. Where the intervention can be viewed as a project the principles of project management can be applied. The science of project management is now relatively mature and a number of well-established tools exist to help project managers including Gantt charts, milestone plans, critical path analysis and risk matrices. The NHS has used a project management methodology known as Projects in Controlled Environments (PRINCE) for a number of years.

PRINCE is a project management method, which was first developed by the Central Computer and Telecommunications Agency (CCTA), and is now, in its current incarnation of PRINCE2, the UK Government's de facto standard for project management in IT[5].

The PRINCE2 methodology describes a set of eight processes: (1) starting up a project; (2) initiating a project; (3) controlling a stage; (4) managing product delivery; (5) managing stage boundaries; (6) closing a project; (7) directing a project; and (8) planning. Each process is made up of a set of activities, each of which is described in a fairly schematic way with a set of inputs and outputs as well as a statement of objectives, an indication of who should be responsible and some guidance on how the activity might be accomplished. A key element in PRINCE2 is the business case, which is not just used to justify the initiation of the project but which also plays a role as a working document throughout the life of the project.

Perspectives on organisational change

PRINCE2 is a straightforward and practical tool designed to help managers accomplish a certain set of tasks, those associated with running projects. The other approaches to change management are, to a greater or a lesser extent, also intended as guides for managers, techniques to help those responsible for running organisations to achieve the changes that they, or their masters, perceive to be necessary. Iles and Sutherland set out to provide a practical guide for working managers. The focus is inevitably on planned, 'programmatic' approaches to change. If one accepts McNulty and Ferlie's conclusions, however, it could be argued that the change on the scale demanded by the IOM cannot be accomplished 'top-down' by managers. Other writers have looked at other perspectives on change. Bate *et al.* ask whether the theories that social and political scientists have used to understand movements for social change might have some application here[6]. The idea is that the kind of 'grass-roots' movements that have successfully effected change in political and environmental campaigns might be able to succeed where the old approaches to reform of health care organisations have often failed. Rather than managers attempting to push through traditional programmes of change, they might seek to foster informal 'communities of practice' through which individuals can work together to achieve ends that they identify for themselves.

The spread of innovation

The same authors contributed to a systematic review of the literature dealing with a related question: the spread of innovation[7]. They distinguish between the formal, planned dissemination of innovation (new behaviours, techniques, ways of working aimed at improving outcomes, efficiency, effectiveness or users' experience) and the diffusion of such innovations through a more complex, organic process that emerges from people's responses to their local situation. They summarise their findings in a complex model that identifies a great many different factors that can help or hinder the spread of an innovation (see Figure 12.1).

A Bayesian model of organisational change

Gustafson *et al.* considered a slightly more restricted set of factors that might predict the success or failure of an organisational change[8]. In a particularly bold initiative, they attempted to establish weights for the various factors that could be expressed as subjective probabilities and build a Bayesian model whose predictions could be tested empirically. A panel was nominated by experts in organisational change. Interviews with members of the panel and a

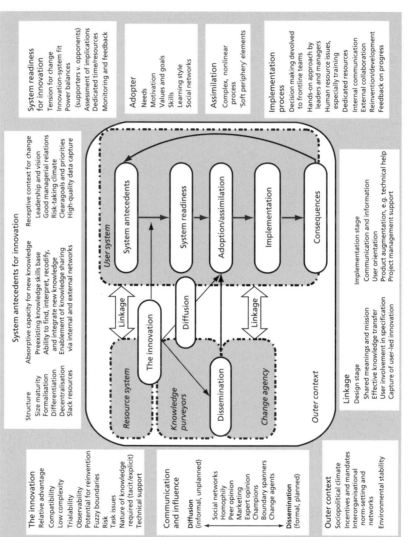

Figure 12.1 Conceptual model for considering the determinants of diffusion, dissemination and implementation in health service delivery. With permission from Greenhalgh T, *et al.* Diffusion of innovations in service organizations. *Milbank Quarterly* 2004; **82:** 581–629.

literature search identified a set of factors that might influence the success of a change project. The panel then met to review these factors and agree on a set of factors to be included in the model. Given that the aim was to develop a Bayesian model, the set of factors identified had to be conditionally independent; they also had to identify criteria that could be used to measure the extent to which a factor was present in a given case. They identified 18 factors:

- the existence of a mandate for change;
- leadership commitment, involvement and support;
- the support of informal opinion leaders;
- middle managers' involvement and support;
- dissatisfaction with existing processes;
- staff involvement and support;
- prior understanding of customers' needs;
- an effective or prestigious change agent;
- external sources of ideas;
- funding;
- relative advantages;
- radicalness of the redesign;
- flexibility of the redesign;
- evidence of effectiveness;
- complexity of implementation plan;
- work environment;
- staff changes required;
- monitoring and feedback.

Each factor could have a high, middle or low rating, which would indicate the extent to which it was at work in a given project.

The experts were then asked to estimate the individual likelihood ratios for each factor, using two methods. Where the methods disagreed, the experts were asked to think again. The experts also had to come up with a figure for the prior probability of a project succeeding. They estimated that a project had 16% of success if it involved changing processes and 5% if it involved cultural change. The finished model was then tested on data from 221 actual projects for which the project leaders (not the expert panel or the authors of the paper but the people who had actually led the projects) gave ratings of low, middle or high for the 18 factors and a judgement of whether or not it had succeeded. The system proved pretty effective, with an area under the receiver operating characteristic (ROC) curve of 0.84. (Note: ROC curves are used to compare tests[9]. They plot the sensitivity against 1 – the specificity at different decision thresholds. When test results are used to inform decision-making, there is always a trade-off between sensitivity and specificity. The optimal balance of false alarms on the one hand and misses on the other will depend on the consequences of these kinds of errors, not on any characteristic of the test. Since ROC curves plot the performance of the test across all possible decision thresholds, the area under the ROC curve is a threshold-independent measure of diagnostic accuracy.) A test that does no better than chance will have an area under the curve of 0.5, one that never makes errors of any sort will have an area under the curve of 1.0, suggesting that the 18 factors identified are the important ones and that estimates obtained for their impact on the final outcome were appropriate. It is an interesting attempt to apply the kinds of quantitative methods described earlier in this book within a field where more qualitative forms of research are the norm.

Conclusion

The aim of health informatics is to improve health care through the improved management of health information. That covers a wide range of change projects. In the next two chapters I look at a number of recent initiatives. I have made a distinction between the use of information and information technology. In Chapter 13, I consider initiatives that have attempted to improve health outcomes through the dissemination of information about best practice. In Chapter 14, I look at projects that make use of IT to enable changes in the organisation of health care, the kind of IT-induced organisational change discussed above.

References

1. Committee on Quality of Health Care in America, Institute of Medicine. *Crossing the Quality Chasm*. Washington, DC: Institute of Medicine, 2001.
2. Venkatraman N. IT-induced business reconfiguration. In: Morton S, ed. *The Corporation of the 1990s*. Oxford: Oxford University Press, 1991.
3. McNulty T, Ferlie E. *Reengineering Healthcare: The Complexities of Organisational Transformation*. Oxford: Oxford University Press, 2002.
4. Iles V, Sutherland K. *Organisational Change: A Review for Health Care Managers, Professionals and Researchers*. London: National Co-ordinating Centre for Service Delivery and Organisation, 2002.
5. Bentley C. *PRINCE2: A Practical Handbook*. Oxford: Butterworth–Heinemann, 2002.
6. Bate P, Robert G, Bevan H. The next phase of healthcare improvement: what can we learn from social movements? *Qual Saf Health Care* 2004;13(1):62–66.
7. Greenhalgh T, Robert G, Macfarlane F, Bate P, Kyriakidou O. Diffusion of innovations in service organizations: systematic review and recommendations. *Milbank Q* 2004;82(4):581–629.
8. Gustafson DH, Sainfort F, Eichler M, Adams L, Bisognano M, Steudel H. Developing and testing a model to predict outcomes of organizational change. *Health Serv Res* 2003;38(2):751–776.
9. Altman D. *Practical Statistics for Medical Research*. London: Chapman & Hall, 1991.

CHAPTER 13
Achieving change through information

The patient journey

When most of us think how health care is delivered – how diagnoses are made and treatments decided upon – the image that comes to mind is probably of a consultation. The context will vary, it might be in a GP's surgery, an outpatient clinic or at the bedside in an acute ward, but the essential idea of this special sort of meeting between doctor and patient is always there. That we think in this way has important consequences for how we organise the delivery of health care. It is a model that assigns a privileged role to the expert physician, who exercises his or her independent judgement in making decisions about individual patients, decisions that then determine what happens to the patient until the next consultation. If we think of a patient's treatment as a journey, the appropriate metaphor might be of a traveller without a map who employs a succession of knowledgeable guides to take him or her to the desired destination.

However, if each of the specialists contributing to the care of a patient acts as an independent authority, there is a danger that an absence of coordination will reduce the quality of care received. To return to the metaphor, it might be more efficient for the traveller's guides to agree the complete itinerary for the journey at the outset, allowing the journey to be planned more effectively. Although in medicine, as with complex travel arrangements, things do not always go according to plan, for many conditions and treatments it is possible to map out a route through the system that will work for a significant number of patients. This is a very different way of thinking about health care, focusing not on the consultation but on the patient's journey through the health care system. We no longer think of the patient's management as shaped by a succession of decisions, each taken independently, but rather as a coordinated attempt to maintain a predetermined trajectory. This way of thinking is increasingly common in attempts to improve the quality of health care by disseminating information.

Berg and Bergen have argued that although each individual patient's trajectory is unique and unpredictable, if we aggregate categories of patients, the proportion of patients that will follow a 'typical' trajectory is sufficiently predictable to be made the basis of clinical thinking[1]. It is therefore possible to organise health services around 'care paths', which make the steps and decisions involved in managing a typical case explicit and facilitate much of the routine work involved in caring for patients. Thinking in terms of care pathways allows for a much greater degree of planning and coordination. They believe that this will radically change patients' experience of health care, reduce waiting times and optimise the use of resources. In support of their argument, they identify a set of logistical principles that, once the idea of care pathways is accepted, can be used to great advantage. They argue that the organising principle used in resource allocation should be the optimisation of patient flows; that the specification of care pathways – including criteria for identifying urgent, routine and non-standard patients – will clarify responsibilities and ensure better coordination of care. The specification in advance of a complete trajectory will mean that downstream constraints, e.g. a shortage of post-operative beds, can be anticipated before any action is initiated. This principle of a planned trajectory should also improve efficiency by ensuring that the necessary preparatory work is undertaken before tasks are initiated.

Imagine a clinical audit revealed that patients referred to a consultant with a certain condition were always, or almost always, re-referred for a particular investigation. Perhaps if the investigation was relatively cheap and fairly safe, it should be ordered by the referring GP so that it could be carried out before the patient sees the consultant. If that would generally be useful but occasionally inappropriate, perhaps the consultant and the referring GPs could agree criteria for when it should be done. The idea is that although patients are, of course, all unique and each must be given individual attention, actually for certain conditions most patients are dealt with in broadly the same way and we can therefore improve the quality of health care that we provide by coordinating the activities of the different professionals involved according to predefined plans.

In fact there is stronger argument than that, if we can establish, from empirical evidence, what is the best way to treat a particular group of patients. Setting out a guideline or protocol for how they should be managed is then not only a tool for improving the efficiency of the process but also a way of ensuring that responsible clinicians comply with best practice. On this argument, some of the variation in how patients are treated stems not from the need to respond to the real differences between patients and their conditions but from variations in the quality of clinical decision-making and the failure of systems to ensure that the best possible care is provided. In the rest of this chapter I look at three initiatives that attempt to disseminate standards for best practice. The first, the National Service Frameworks (NSFs), is an example of an attempt by government to impose a universal standard for the treatment of certain common conditions. The second, Integrated Care Pathways (ICPs), is a technique whereby a multidisciplinary group agrees a local standard for the management of a particular category of patients. The third, Clinical Guidelines, deals with the more general idea of standardised plans for patient management.

National Service Frameworks

In 1998 the Department of Health in England initiated a rolling programme of standards, termed NSFs, for the management of the major diseases and health problems. Starting with coronary heart disease and cancer, at the time of writing, frameworks have published for paediatric intensive care, mental health, older people, diabetes, long-term conditions, renal services and children. The NSFs are lengthy, comprehensive documents produced by 'expert reference groups'; they set out national standards for levels of care (what should be done), models of service provision (how it should be done) and targets against which performance is to be judged.

The NSF for coronary heart disease sets out standards for improving the prevention of the disease in the population in general and separate standards for prevention in high-risk groups[2]. For example, one standard states that GPs should identify all people at a significant risk of coronary heart disease and offer them appropriate advice and treatment to reduce their risk. Target levels are defined for blood pressure and cholesterol. Other standards cover the investigation and treatment of acute and chronic heart conditions. The framework sets out quite specific targets by which the performance of hospitals and primary care organisations is to be judged, and these include standards to do with informatics, for the recording and organisation of patient data: 'the primary care team should have all medical records and correspondence held in a way that allows them to be retrieved readily in date order'. The NSF sets out criteria for key investigations and treatments, and goals for maximum waiting times. So, for example, patients with evidence of continuing extensive ischaemia (a strongly positive exercise test) or persistent angina are to be offered angiography and should have to wait no longer than 6 months for the investigation.

The NHS Cancer Plan, which is taken to be the NSF for cancer, was similar[3]. It contained commitments for maximum waiting times for patients who, in the opinion of their GP, were suffering from suspected cancer. Guidelines that set out, quite precisely, who was and who was not to be seen under the urgent referral rule were later published[4]. So, for example, the guidelines dealing with childhood tumours include the rule that children are to be referred for an urgent appointment if they are suffering from a 'headache of recent origin with two or more of the following features: increasing in severity or frequency, noted to be worse in the morning or causing early awakening, associated with vomiting, associated with neurological signs (squint, ataxia), associated with behavioural change or deterioration in school performance'.

Impact of National Service Frameworks

The publication of the frameworks generated a great deal of attention, and a number of papers and letters appeared expressing anxiety about their implications for workload. Hippisley-Cox and Pringle considered the impact of the requirement in the Coronary Health Disease NSF that GPs identify all patients with established coronary heart disease or stroke, record their coronary risk factors, offer appropriate treatment, and identify and treat patients at high risk of developing coronary heart disease[5]. They estimated that in an average practice of 10 000 patients about 904 items would have to be recorded and about 2221 disease control measures would be required.

In 2005 the Department of Health published a progress report that highlighted significant areas of progress and concluded that the NSF was making a real difference for patients, noting, for example, that there were no longer patients waiting over 6 months for heart surgery[6]. Majeed *et al.* assessed the impact of the NSF for coronary heart disease on the management of the disease in primary care and found generally positive results when practice was compared to the defined standards[7]. Key risk factors were being recorded, there were high rates of uptake for influenza immunisation and higher than previously reported rates for the use of angiotensin-converting enzyme (ACE) inhibitors. The most significant failure recorded was that few patients seemed to have had an ECG, the gold standard investigation in the diagnosis of heart disease. The shortage of equipment and trained personnel to perform key investigations is also noted in progress reports for the National Cancer Plan[8]. A small qualititative study by Checkland suggested that although primary care staff were supportive of NSFs in principle, in practice the frameworks had relatively little impact, with only 6% of staff having read the full document and only 31% the summary[9]. None of the three practices studied had a plan for the implementation of any of the NSFs.

The conclusion seems to be that NSFs can be successful in effecting certain kinds of organisational change, for example, where a clearly specified change is mandated and the resources required to make the change are available. There are, however, limits to their effectiveness when it comes to changing the behaviour of individual practitioners. The NSFs represent an extreme of the top-down centralised approach to management that McNulty and Ferlie noted was often unsuccessful as an approach to change in the public sector. The next section deals with a very different approach, in which guidelines are agreed locally by teams of co-workers. First I want to make an observation about the operation of the 2-week referral rule introduced in the National Cancer Plan, partly because it reveals an interesting consequence of setting targets for waiting times and partly because it makes use of a piece of probability theory that I would like at least to mention in passing.

Fast tracking appointments
A great deal of attention has been focused on the consequences of the 2-week referral rule. This target has generally been met, with 98.5% of patients with suspected cancer being seen within 2 weeks[10]. Whether or not the rule has had a beneficial impact on outcomes is less clear. Since the demand for appointments fluctuates, availability can only be guaranteed if the maximum

capacity is greater than the average demand, if there is spare capacity. We can use techniques from probability theory to determine how much spare capacity is required to give, for example, a 99% guarantee that appointments will be available. The number of events that occur in a fixed time interval can be modelled using a Poisson distribution: if events happen at a rate of μ events per interval, the probability that no more than r events will happen in the given interval is

$$\sum_{k=0}^{r} \frac{e^{-\mu}\mu^{r}}{r!}$$

This is a standard function in spreadsheets making it easy to work out, for example, that a clinic that usually receives 24 patients will have to be able to cope with 36 patients in order to meet demand 99% of the time, and that 50% spare capacity is therefore required. Operating a waiting list, of course, makes it easier to cope with fluctuations in demand, but the shorter the waiting list, the less scope it allows. Thomas *et al.* showed that, for most clinics, an excess capacity of two patient slots per clinic was required to operate the 2-week referral rule[11]. In general, subdividing a group of patients and fast tracking some of them will have the effect of increasing waiting times for the group as a whole. For the tactic to have a positive impact on overall outcomes, therefore, there must be a real difference in the two subgroups so that the benefits of fast tracking one outweigh the cost of making the other wait.

Integrated Care Pathways

The National Pathways Association offers the following definition of ICPs: 'An Integrated Care Pathway determines locally agreed multidisciplinary practice, based on guidelines and evidence where available, for a specific patient/client group. It forms all or part of the clinical record, documents the care given and facilitates the evaluation of outcomes for continuous quality improvement'[12].

The thinking behind ICPs can be traced back to the use of critical path planning and process mapping in industry, techniques that date from the 1950s. In the 1980s, clinicians in the USA began to develop the idea of pathways, then termed Anticipated Recovery Pathways, in order to meet the requirements of Health Management Organisations and the insurance industry. By 1994, the Anticipated Recovery Pathway had evolved, in the UK, into the Integrated Care Pathway. The NeLH Pathways Database was launched in 2002 to enable the free sharing of ICPs and ICP Projects across the UK.

Integrated Care Pathways in stroke

Consider, as an example, the use of ICPs in the management of stroke. A stroke is a sudden episode in which the flow of blood interferes with the normal functioning of the brain. There are different ways in which this can happen. In cerebral haemorrhage, the problem is caused by bleeding into or around the brain; in cerebral thrombosis it is caused by blockage of blood vessels in the brain, usually because of a blood clot. In a subarachnoid haemorrhage, blood from an artery close to the brain surface leaks into the space between the membranes that cover the brain and spinal chord. Strokes affect 1 in 500 persons and occur mainly in the elderly. Although stroke is the third most common cause of death in developed countries, strokes vary greatly in severity. The management of stroke patients is essentially a matter of rehabilitation, of helping the patient to recover as much as possible of normal function and to cope with any permanent impairments or disabilities. Dedicated stroke units exist to bring together the different specialists that this requires. In 1995 a stroke unit was opened at the Charing Cross Hospital in London, and an ICP for stroke was developed for the unit[13].

The multidisciplinary team dealing with a stroke patient includes a doctor, pharmacist, dietitian, occupational therapist, nurse, physiotherapist, speech therapist and social worker. The development of the ICP brought together representatives of the different groups. The ICP was developed with reference to both the published evidence on best practice and the constraints of the local situation through a process that was managed by a core team of a consultant and two ICP coordinators. Three specially convened meetings of the multidisciplinary team were required before the draft ICP could be agreed.

The resulting ICP is, in concrete terms, a document. It is set out as a grid with a column for each day covered by the ICP (the team decided to restrict the ICP to cover only the week after admission and the 2 weeks leading up to discharge, since those were the periods where care could most easily be standardized and where the need for coordination was greatest). There is a section to be completed and signed by each member of the team. The pathway does not specify in detail every action to be performed in every case but the principle categories of assessment are set out and the appropriate treatments and management options indicated. The ICP also indicates the targets that define good quality care for the condition: the avoidance of bedsores, chest infections and deep vein thrombosis, so that the document can be used to audit performance against those standards. One of the most important elements of the ICP is the recording of variances. Inevitably there will be patients whose care does not follow the usual trajectory. The designers of the ICP must, naturally, ensure that data is recorded about these patients and the circumstances, which meant that the ICP could not be applied. Such variances can reveal problems in the way care is delivered or shortcomings in the ICP.

The ICP was introduced when the stroke unit opened. All staff were given training in the use of ICP and a poster was put up in the staff coffee room to remind staff how the ICP document was to be filled in. A paper written after a 4-month pilot period reports a positive response to the ICP but makes it clear that medical staff failed to complete all the sections of the document and that many of the 13 patients treated during the pilot period had had to be taken off the ICP at some point. The ICP proved inflexible.

For and against Integrated Care Pathways

The evidence surrounding the use of ICPs in stroke is, perhaps surprisingly, negative. A before–after study found some evidence of an improvement in certain aspects of care (fewer urinary tract infections)[14]. An RCT involving 152 patients found no significant differences in the processes of interdisciplinary coordination and patient management between patients managed according to an ICP and patients in a control group[15]. The ICP was associated with various positive outcomes (greater uptake of stroke-specific assessments, better documentation of rehabilitation goals, improved communication between patients' carers and primary care physicians) and some negative outcomes (smaller proportion of patients having goals for higher-level functioning and worse awareness of carers' needs). The conclusion seems to be that stroke units that already feature specialised multidisciplinary input may not derive a great benefit from ICPs. The research led some authorities to suggest that recovery from stroke is too variable a process for ICPs to be applicable[16].

It does not follow from this that they are a bad idea, but rather that the impact will not always be wholly positive. There are many different ways in which we can try to improve the efficiency of an organisation; ICPs represent one approach to changing the way we organise health care services and should be considered as an option where change is likely to lead to improvements.

Clinical guidelines

ICPs are just one initiative that attempts to introduce normative clinical guidelines. The use of clinical guidelines is now widely established as a way of promoting best practice. A recent systematic review found considerable evidence that the dissemination and implementation of clinical guidelines improved compliance with recommended practices. However, there was a considerable variation in the size of the observed effects and most studies reported only modest or moderate improvements in care[17]. One of the more controversial topics that has been made the subject of clinical guidelines is the management of hypertension.

Treating hypertension according to clinical guidelines

Targets for identifying and treating patients with high blood pressure formed part of the NSF for coronary heart disease. There have, however, been other initiatives. The British Hypertension Society published a guideline for the management of hypertension in March 2004[18]. Another, from the National Institute for Clinical Excellence, appeared in August 2004[19]. The guidelines

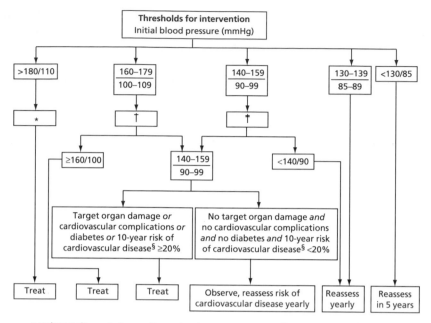

<table>
<tr><td colspan="5">**Thresholds for intervention**
Initial blood pressure (mmHg)</td></tr>
</table>

Figure 13.1 The BHS hypertension guideline. From [18] with permission from the BMJ Publishing Group.

The figure shows a flow chart with the following elements:

Thresholds for intervention — Initial blood pressure (mmHg), branching to: >180/110; 160–179 / 100–109; 140–159 / 90–99; 130–139 / 85–89; <130/85.

>180/110 → * → Treat

160–179 / 100–109 → † → ≥160/100 → Treat; or 140–159 / 90–99 →

140–159 / 90–99 → ‡ → <140/90

140–159 / 90–99 branches into:
- Target organ damage *or* cardiovascular complications *or* diabetes *or* 10-year risk of cardiovascular disease§ ≥20% → Treat
- No target organ damage *and* no cardiovascular complications *and* no diabetes *and* 10-year risk of cardiovascular disease§ <20% → Observe, reassess risk of cardiovascular disease yearly

130–139 / 85–89 → Reassess yearly

<130/85 → Reassess in 5 years

* Unless malignant phase of hypertensive emergency, confirm over 1–2 weeks then treat

† If cardiovascular complications, target organ damage, or diabetes is present, confirm over 3–4 weeks then treat; if absent, remeasure weekly and treat if blood pressure persists at these levels over 4–12 weeks

‡ If cardiovascular complications, target organ damage, or diabetes is present, confirm over 12 weeks then treat; if absent, remeasure monthly and treat if these levels are maintained and if estimated 10-year cardiovascular disease risk is ≥20%

§ Assessed with risk chart for cardiovascular disease

specify how blood pressure is to be measured, how hypertensive patients should be evaluated, and define treatment goals in the form of 'target' blood pressures. At the core of, for example, the British Hypertension Society guideline is a flow chart, shown in Figure 13.1, which specifies treatment thresholds and target blood pressures.

The publication of these documents generated a certain amount of resentment, with GPs complaining about the fact that there are multiple sources of guidance, and that the guidelines were long and complex and changes from previous guidelines seemed unjustified[20].

Researchers looking at compliance with earlier guidelines – and a number have been published by various national and international bodies – have generally reported low compliance. GPs often seem to adopt pragmatic thresholds for initiating treatment that are less aggressive than those specified in the guidelines[21]. One study found 'adequate' awareness of the content of a guideline in only 19% of GPs[22]. The question of whether or not practitioners 'comply' with guidelines seems, in the eyes of some observers, to reflect an inappropriate prescriptive approach to the dissemination of such materials. Researchers have found that patient preferences for treatment can be at odds with the targets given in the guidelines[23]. Others have reported that the recommended treatments were contraindicated in as many as half the patients managed in primary care[24].

The key issue is not whether guidelines can be effective, but how they can be implemented so that they can be most effective. There are many pitfalls. If there are too many guidelines, they will fail to command attention. If they are too detailed, users may consider them long-winded and overcomplicated. If they are too general, they will often not be applicable. Getting the balance right will be a matter of judgement and will depend on the problem being addressed and the context in which the guideline is to be applied. One approach, which solves some but not all of the above difficulties, is to incorporate the guideline into a computer system.

Computerised guidelines

In recent years, it has become apparent that active management of blood glucose levels can help improve outcomes for ICU patients. One unit, in response to this finding, introduced a guideline for glucose regulation[25]. Patients in the ICU were randomly assigned to be managed either by a nurse using a paper version of the guideline or a nurse who received automated alerts via the ICU's computer system, which incorporated a computerised form of the guideline. Interestingly, the management received by patients managed according to the computerised guideline was significantly better.

A number of groups are currently working on the development of formalisms, which allow the succinct representation of more complex protocols. Fox *et al.* have developed a language that allows protocols to be defined in terms of a small set of generic entities (tasks, actions, plans, decisions, enquiries) and a graphical editor that allows clinicians rapidly to specify a protocol in terms that can be translated into a computerised representation[26]. An example of Proforma's graphical notation is shown in Figure 13.2. The Proforma language is intended to be used with a suite of tools that enable the rapid publication of guidelines as 'Publets' – small interactive web-based applications. Once the technology has been developed that will allow these kinds of tools to be used to provide large numbers of guidelines integrated with the software used to store patient data, the potential for guideline-based decision support ought to be enormous. Nevertheless, it is worth sounding a note of caution. Guidelines to support prescribing have already, for some years, been incorporated into electronic patient record systems and, although there is evidence that this can improve prescribing, there is also evidence of difficulties.

Prescribing guidelines

One way of getting prescribing guidelines into practice is via systems that are designed to automate the medication ordering process. These systems, known

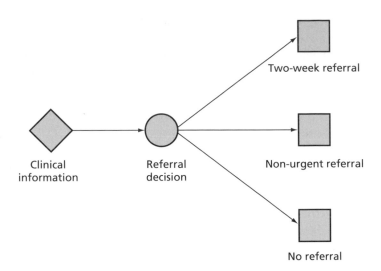

Figure 13.2 A simple Proforma guideline. Reproduced with permission, © OpenClinical.

as computerised physician order entry (CPOE) systems, are advocated primarily as the way to cut prescription errors. Clinical guidelines are built into almost all CPOE systems, sometimes providing advice on doses, routes and frequencies, and sometimes checking for known allergies or other counterindications. Advocates argue that such systems can substantially enhance the quality of care and improve patient safety[27]. A systematic review of CPOE found evidence of a significant reduction in medication error rates and evidence of an impact on costs and quality[28]. The conclusion was that the known benefits of CPOE justified their introduction but certain specific questions about the systems need to be addressed: what, for example, are the factors that determine when systems will succeed? The good news has to be tempered with an awareness that introducing CPOE requires a high degree of organisational change as well as a substantial upfront investment both in terms of the financial cost of buying or implementing a system and in terms of redesigning processes to accommodate the system. As with any new and complex computer system, there is also a potential for introducing errors, reducing rather than enhancing safety. One study in the review found that incorrect default dosing or route suggestions led to potentially erroneous orders.

It turns out, when you look in detail at the kinds of prescribing mistakes that are made, that there are lots of different factors to consider, and the most important is medical knowledge. According to Bobb *et al.* over 60% of mistakes are attributed to inadequate medical knowledge[29]. Their data also suggest that although CPOE can be highly effective at intercepting mistakes, only the most sophisticated versions of it are effective at reducing the important mistakes. Half the 'clinically significant' prescribing errors were only rated as 'possibly preventable' with CPOE. They concluded that 'a CPOE system with advanced computer-based decision support should deliver specific recommendations by matching individual patient characteristics to a computerised knowledge base'. This, however, is hard and most commercial CPOE systems do not address this. There is a further problem with generating these kinds of recommendations. Weingart *et al.* looked at a CPOE system in primary care and found that physicians overrode 91.2% of drug allergy and 89.4% of high-severity drug interaction alerts[30]. Yet there were few adverse drug events. A review of the alerts found that 36.5% were inappropriate. They concluded that a system that generates too many alerts will be ignored.

Fernando *et al.* looked at the safety features of four prescribing systems used in the UK, none of which implemented all of the safety features that an expert panel deemed important[31]. For example, none of the systems warned against prescribing aspirin to a child of 8. All failed to alert the user of the possible confusion when prescribing one of two drugs with similar names.

Conclusions

One of the grand challenges identified for health informatics in Part 1 was the development of systems to improve clinicians' access to knowledge. A number of initiatives, reviewed in this chapter, have attempted to improve the quality of health care, not so much by improving access to knowledge as by actively disseminating information about best practice. The onus is less on the practitioner to keep up to date and more on the system. This may seem a slight shift of emphasis, but it is an important one. It leads to a conception of the problem where the issue is not one of professional education but of behaviour modification. Many so-called decision support systems are not tools designed to help clinicians make sense of complex problems but, rather, automated reminders that tell him or her what to do and when[32]. Such systems, as shown in some of the research summarised above, are not without difficulties. The problem is getting the balance right: telling people what they need to know when they need to know it, without creating systems that are intrusive, offering non-specific, inappropriate or unwanted advice.

References

1. Berg M, Bergen C. Meeting the challenge: integrating quality improvement and patient care information systems. In: Berg M, ed. *Health Information Management*. New York: Routledge, 2004.
2. Department of Health. *National Service Framework for Coronary Heart Disease*. London: Department of Health, 2000.
3. Department of Health. *The NHS Cancer Plan: A Plan for Investment, a Plan for Reform*. London: Department of Health, 2000.
4. Department of Health. *Referral Guidelines for Suspected Cancer*. Health Service Circular (HSC) 2000/013, 2000.

5. Hippisley-Cox J, Pringle M. General practice workload implications of the National Service Framework for Coronary Heart Disease: cross-sectional survey. *BMJ* 2001;323(7307):269–270.

6. DH Coronary Heart Disease Policy Team. *Leading the Way Progress Report 2005: The Coronary Heart Disease National Service Framework*. London: Department of Health Publications, 2005.

7. Majeed A, Williams J, de Lusignan S, Chan T. Management of heart failure in primary care after implementation of the National Service Framework for Coronary Heart Disease: a cross-sectional study. *Public Health* 2005;119(2):105–111.

8. Commission for Health Improvement. *National Service Framework Assessments No. 1: NHS Cancer Care in England and Wales*. England: Commission for Health Improvement, 2001.

9. Checkland K. National Service Frameworks and UK general practitioners: street-level bureaucrats at work? *Social Health Illness* 2004;26(7):951–975.

10. NHS. *The NHS Cancer Plan Three Year Progress Report: Maintaining the Momentum*. London: Department of Health Publications, 2003.

11. Thomas SJ, Williams MV, Burnet NG, Baker CR. How much surplus capacity is required to maintain low waiting times? *Clin Oncol* 2001;13(1):24–28.

12. National Electronic Library for Health About Integrated Care Pathways (ICPs). http://libraries.nelh.nhs.uk/pathways/aboutICPs.asp (accessed on 25 May 2005).

13. Brereton J. Pathways for stroke care. In: Johnson S, ed. *Pathways of Care*. Oxford: Blackwell Science, 1997.

14. Kwan J, Hand P, Dennis M, Sandercock P. Effects of introducing an integrated care pathway in an acute stroke unit. *Age Ageing* 2004;33(4):362–367.

15. Sulch D, Evans A, Melbourn A, Kalra L. Does an integrated care pathway improve processes of care in stroke rehabilitation? A randomized controlled trial. *Age Ageing* 2002;31:175–179.

16. Kwan J, Sandercock P. In-hospital care pathways for stroke. *Cochrane Database Syst Rev* 2004;18(4).

17. Grimshaw JM, Thomas RE, MacLennan G, *et al*. Effectiveness and efficiency of guideline dissemination and implementation strategies. *Health Technol Assess* 2004;8(6):iii–iv, 1–72.

18. Williams B, Poulter NR, Brown MJ, *et al*. BHS guidelines working party, for the British Hypertension Society. British Hypertension Society guidelines for hypertension management 2004 (BHS-IV): summary. *BMJ* 2004;328(7440):634–640.

19. Hebert K. NICE sets out guidelines for hypertension. *BMJ* 2004;329(7464):475.

20. Campbell NC, Murchie P. Treating hypertension with guidelines in general practice. *BMJ* 2004;329(7465):523–524.

21. Frijling BD, Spies TH, Lobo CM, Hulscher ME, van Drenth BB, Braspenning JC, Prins A, van der Wouden JC, Grol RP. Blood pressure control in treated hypertensive patients: clinical performance of general practitioners. *Br J Gen Pract* 2001;51(462):9–14.

22. Hagemeister J, Schneider CA, Barabas S, Schadt R, Wassmer G, Mager G, Pfaff H, Hopp HW. Hypertension guidelines and their limitations – the impact of physicians' compliance as evaluated by guideline awareness. *J Hypertens* 2001;19(11):2079–2086.

23. Montgomery AA, Harding J, Fahey T. Shared decision making in hypertension: the impact of patient preferences on treatment choice. *Fam Pract* 2001;18(3):309–313.

24. Spence JD, Hurley TC, Spence JD. Actual practice in hypertension: implications for persistence with and effectiveness of therapy. *Curr Hypertens Rep* 2001;3(6):481–487.

25. Rood E, Bosman RJ, van der Spoel JI, Taylor P, Zandstra DF. Use of a computerized guideline for glucose regulation in the intensive care unit improved both guideline adherence and glucose regulation. *J Am Med Inform Assoc* 2005;12(2):172–180.

26. Sutton DR, Fox J. The syntax and semantics of the PROforma guideline modeling language. *J Am Med Inform Assoc* 2003;10(5):433–443.

27. Kuperman GJ, Gibson RF. Computer physician order entry: benefits, costs, and issues. *Ann Intern Med* 2003;139(1):31–39.

28. Kaushal R, Shojania KG, Bates DW. Effects of computerized physician order entry and clinical decision support systems on medication safety. *Arch Intern Med* 2003;163:1409–1416.

29. Bobb A, Gleason K, Husch M, Feinglass J, Yarnold PR, Noskin GA. The epidemiology of prescribing errors: the potential impact of computerized prescriber order entry. *Arch Intern Med* 2004;164(7):785–792.

30. Weingart SN, Toth M, Sands DZ, Aronson MD, Davis RB, Phillips RS. Physicians' decisions to override computerized drug alerts in primary care. *Arch Intern Med* 2003;163:2625–2631.

31. Fernando B, Savelyich BS, Avery AJ, Sheikh A, Bainbridge M, Horsfield P, Teasdale S. Prescribing safety features of general practice computer systems: evaluation using simulated test cases. *BMJ* 2004;328(7449):1171–1172.

32. Garg AX, Adhikari NK, McDonald H, *et al.* Effects of computerized clinical decision support systems on practitioner performance and patient outcomes: a systematic review. *JAMA* 2005;293(10):1223–1238.

CHAPTER 14

Achieving change through information technology

IT and organisational change in the NHS

Implementing a programme of organisational change will have a wide range of effects, including many that will not have been anticipated. Plans normally have to be adapted to take account of changing circumstances. Both the process of change and the outcomes will often be viewed differently by the different groups involved. Given this complexity, it is inevitably impossible to look at the research and identify a single framework or theory of change that is the 'right one'. Iles and Sutherland highlight a number of important factors: a structured approach – e.g. one based on a critical review of the available models of change, staff involvement, responsive leadership, avoiding jargon and openness to unanticipated outcomes[1].

The idea that a topic such as organisational change or change management is an important part of health informatics is relatively new. It has, however, very quickly become a mainstream viewpoint. The NHS National Programme for IT, Connecting for Health, acknowledges that its success is dependent upon the successful implementation of a change programme. In the following two sections I review two of the major components of the programme and consider both their implications for organisational change and the role of health informatics research.

Booked admissions

The idea of booked admissions is a simple one. Instead of being put on a waiting list and then being sent notice of an appointment date, patients and their doctors agree an admission date as soon as it is decided that treatment is required. This gives the patients a degree of choice about when they are treated, and also a greater sense of involvement in the decision and reduced uncertainty about the process. Like a lot of simple ideas, however, it is hard to make it work. Introducing booked admissions requires that physicians make commitments further ahead than they otherwise would; it therefore involves a change in working practices, and it also has implications for capacity.

The brief history of booked admissions in the UK involves a maelstrom of agencies, initiatives and improvement programmes. Perhaps the most important event in the story is the publication in 2000 of the *NHS Plan*, a proposal for the 'modernisation' of the NHS[2]. Two features of the plan were seen to be crucial in achieving the desired improvements: the redesign of services around patients and increased patient choice. The Department of Health had already set up the National Patient's Access Team (NPAT) in an attempt to tackle the problem of over-long waiting lists. The NPAT launched a National Booked Admissions Programme (NBAP) with the aim of making access to care more convenient. The Cancer Services Collaborative (CSC) was set up as part of the NBAP to look at the particular problems associated with the organisation of cancer services in the UK. The CSC followed a set of strategies proposed by a US think tank, the Institute for Healthcare Improvement (IHI). Phase 1 of the NBAP ran from November 1999 to March 2001. The programme became part of the NHS Modernisation Agency in April 2001 and at the time of writing is the responsibility of the National Programme for IT, Connecting for Health, having changed its name first to the National Booking Team and then to Choose and Book.

The IHI proposes a model for improvement[3]. According to the model, the team charged with achieving improvement must ask three questions: What are we trying to accomplish? How will we know that a change is an improvement? What change can we make that will result in an improvement? The answers to these questions are used to set goals. Progress towards goals is made through a process of 'plan, do, study, act' cycles, making the approach an example of the action research paradigm outlined in Chapter 12. The focus is on small changes that can be implemented and tested in 1 or 2 weeks. The IHI argues that real change requires changing the system. It is not enough just to try a bit harder to make the existing system work better, we have to alter the system; the best way of achieving that, according to the IHI, is through incremental improvements. The CSC set up a series of pilot projects that were asked to employ the IHI methodology in four strategy areas: connect up the patient journey, develop the team around the patient journey, make the patient experience central to the journey and ensure capacity at each stage of the journey. Although booked admissions are seen as central to the implementation of the NHS plan and an important part of the mission of the CSC and the Modernisation Agency, other ways of improving the patient journey were considered.

In an article in the *BMJ*, members of the CSC reported that teams tested 4400 changes between August 1999 and September 2000[4]. It was found that 65% of projects showed at least a 50% reduction in time to first treatment. Changes improved patient flow and access. For example, patients with suspected bowel cancer in Leicestershire had previously had separate visits for flexible sigmoidoscopy, barium enema and a consultation; this was changed so that all three could be done in a single day. In mid-Anglia radiologists started to refer patients with signs of cancer directly to a chest physician, cutting the patient journey time from 24 days to 11 days[5]. The percentage of patients given booked admissions was 56% for both first outpatient appointment and first diagnostic test, and 62% for first definitive treatment. In another report, a CSC team found that introducing booked admissions for barium enema reduced 'did not attend' (DNA) rates from 10–15% to around 3%, allowing a significant increase in the efficiency with which appointments lists were managed, which would be expected to lower waiting times.

An external evaluation of the work of the NPAT found that at 24 pilot sites the percentage of patients given a booked 'to come in' date increased from 51.7% to 72.7% from March 1999 to March 2000 and then fell again to 66.2% by the end of March 2001[6]. Similarly the proportion of patient waiting over 6 months fell from 10.9% to 10.5% and then rose to 11.9%. DNA rates also fell from 5.7% to 3.1% and then rose to 4%. Most of the improvements made were not sustained. The evaluation also found that the experience of the pilots varied: some pilots were able to achieve considerable improvements, whereas in others the data suggested that the problems only got worse during the period of study.

Implementing booked admissions

A survey of project managers in the various booked admissions pilots indicated that a variety of factors hindered the introduction of booked admissions[7]. These included lack of capacity, lengthening waiting lists, problems recruiting staff, Trust mergers and an increased tendency for patients to change their appointments. Consultants were also blamed: they were said to be reluctant to give up their freedom to determine relative priority and unwilling to plan leave sufficiently far ahead to allow bookings to be made and honoured. The best performing sites were found to be those with effective leadership by both chief executives and senior clinicians.

The authors of the evaluation made four conclusions. First, that in any improvement programme of this kind, there is an awkward balance between leadership from the government and its agencies, working from the top-down and the commitment of the staff on the ground, working from the bottom-up. It is seen as difficult to impose change from the top-down in the health care organisations staffed by professionals whose primary responsibility is to their patients, not their employer. Second, that action is required at different levels, if change is to be achieved. Quality improvement programmes must stimulate change by systems, organisations, teams and individuals. Third, the pilot programmes were considered to have underestimated the time required for changes to take hold. The evidence gathered in the evaluation strongly suggested that improvements were made but not sustained. In part, this was because the programme made available extra funds, which were used to buy additional capacity; once the programme funding was exhausted, this capacity had to be relinquished and this reduced the scope for booking admissions. Fourth, that staff affected by the improvement programme should be able to see that they, as well as patients, can benefit from the changes.

Choice and capacity

One of the problems with the pilot booked admissions programmes was that where existing capacity was stretched, the proportion of appointments that could be offered as booked admissions tended to be reduced. One of the principal arguments in favour of booked admissions is that it will reduce DNA rates and therefore enable the more efficient use of existing appointment slots. Booked admissions are therefore proposed as a way of dealing with the problem of limited capacity. However, it is not as simple as that. Under a conventional system a patient seeing their GP in March might be told in June that their appointment would be in July. With booked admissions the requirement is that the GP seeing the patient in March must be able to say with confidence when the next suitable appointment slot is, which presumably – at least when the programme starts – will be some time in July. But the variability in hospital lengths of stay, emergency admissions and patient-initiated cancellations means that it is not possible to guarantee availability as far ahead as that unless there is considerable spare capacity. Just how much spare capacity is required can be estimated by building mathematical models to estimate the probability distribution of demand for beds.

One such model was developed by Utley *et al.* and tested with real data from the cardiac surgery department at St George's Hospital in London[8]. Their calculations suggest that a typical cardiac surgery department operating with 20% reserve capacity (i.e. 36 beds for an expected demand of 30 beds) would face a crisis of provision roughly on 5% of days. A similar modelling exercise applied to the demand for post-operative intensive care following cardiac surgery suggests that a reserve capacity of 30% would be required to keep the risk of operational overload below 5%[9]. This is a much greater level of spare capacity than is currently available and would be difficult to finance, intensive care beds being one of the most expensive parts of a hospital.

Choose and Book

The Booked Admissions Programme has now evolved into Choose and Book, which will allow GPs to book patients' hospital appointments online during a consultation with the patient. This, clearly, is a significant development, which requires the hospitals to make available data about their appointment lists and also requires hospital consultants both to concede a significant degree of control over their working lives and to delegate a clinically important role, assigning priorities for appointments, to GPs. This in itself would make the initiative a bold one but it goes further in two respects. A central element in the programme, as reflected in the change of name, is the idea of patient choice. From December 2005 all patients are to be offered a choice of 4–5 hospitals or other providers once a GP decides that a referral is required. This, clearly, has a further impact on capacity as some beds will have to be set aside for choices that are not used. The programme also goes further than the Booked Admissions Programme in that patients are to be allowed to make bookings via a call centre to be known as the Booking Management Service.

We can identify three different categories of challenge to be met if this is to be achieved. The first is that the commissioning arrangements, whereby Primary Care Trusts agree contracts with the Secondary Care Trusts to which their GPs refer patients, will have to change to allow the required level of choice. The organisations that commission care and those that provide care will have to come together to agree a Directory of Services (DoS) from which patients in a community can choose. The second is that the booking processes will have to be redesigned. The roles and responsibilities of the referring GP and the consultant shift somewhat with the move to booked admissions. One of the important areas here is the development of booking guidance so that GPs and other booking staff (e.g. those working in the call centre) can ensure that patients are referred appropriately. A significant degree of cooperation between primary and secondary clinicians will be required for this to work. Finally, if anything is to happen, the IT systems that underpin the activity must be designed and built.

Health informatics and booked admissions

The project is ambitious. It involves radical change and could significantly enhance patients' experience of the referral process. The most obvious difficulties though are not really to do with health informatics. The major challenge is in the scale of organisational transformation that is required in order to take advantage of the technology. This involves significant change both in coordinating the activities of Trusts within each local health economy to allow a menu of choices to be provided and in redefining the responsibilities of GPs and hospital consultants, so that the former now control access to clinics run by the latter.

Nevertheless, there are many aspects of the project to which health informatics can contribute, and where the kinds of challenges we have discussed in this book come into play. The redesign of the referral process that is envisaged by booked admissions needs to have a basis in evidence that in turn will be enhanced by careful and appropriate measurement of, for example, waiting times. Similarly if patients are to make informed choices about the providers to whom they can be referred, they need to have access to information derived from data about performance. So we need to turn raw data about Trust performance into the information that patients want. If GPs are to refer appropriately, referral guidelines, which should include criteria for distinguishing between urgent and routine referrals, must be agreed between the GP and the consultant. One area where the issues discussed in this book are particularly apparent is the creation of a DoS.

Compiling a Directory of Service

One of the key steps in delivering the booked admissions programme is the complication of a DoS[10]. This is intended to be a list of all the services available in the NHS. It should be clear that an initiative that is to allow services to be booked electronically needs to have an up-to-date database of what services there are. But, as often happens in health informatics, a simple and apparently straightforward requirement conceals a measure of complexity. One would want the concept of 'service' embodied in the DoS to correspond to that used in the Patient Administration Systems (PAS), which Trusts use to keep track of appointments. Maintaining accurate and up-to-date information in the DoS is only realistic if there is a mapping between the way clinics are represented in a Trust's systems and the way they are represented in the DoS, so that any update in the PAS can automatically be reflected in the DoS. But, at present, the concept of a 'service' required by the DoS is not well defined outside the DoS and will be represented in different ways in different PAS implementations. Clinics are defined in a variety of ways: sometimes, for example, with a named consultant, sometimes not. Often the PAS will identify each clinic with a unique code and a more lengthy description, the PAS software will then arrange that the user is presented with the description and not required to identify the clinic by the code. However, neither the code nor the description will necessarily be appropriate identifiers to represent the clinic in the DoS.

What is needed is a well-defined concept of 'service' that includes all the data items required by the DoS. The problem is that if the DoS implementers come up with such a definition and then expect individual Trusts to provide a mapping from their PAS implementation to the DoS definition of a service, they might be, in effect, requiring Trusts to redesign their systems. At the very least, it is clear that the information in the PAS will have to be reviewed to ensure that clinics and appointment slots can be matched with the services.

In effect, Choose and Book is creating a new system and also a requirement for a level of interoperability between the new system and the old systems. This requirement for interoperability is exactly the issue that the developers of HL7 seek to address.

Electronic transfer of prescriptions

Over the years many authorities have argued for the introduction of electronic prescribing as means of improving the safety and efficiency of the prescribing process. The term 'electronic prescribing' is however ambiguous; the Electronic Prescribing Initiative distinguishes six different levels of electronic prescribing[11]. It suggests that at the most basic level, the term could be taken to refer to a prescribing system that allowed reference to electronic sources of information about drugs. More sophisticated than this would be a stand-alone prescription writer, which allowed users to search by drug name and create a prescription. Such stand-alone systems are obviously less useful than systems in which supporting patient data can be accessed, to allow allergy checks, for example. Systems with this kind of functionality are now relatively common in primary care. We are concerned, in this chapter, with the next three levels of the pyramid, which allow, first, the user to check the prescription against the patient's medication history; second, connectivity between physicians, pharmacists and other agencies; and third, full integration with a medical record.

As many as 649 million prescriptions were generated in 2003–2004, and the figure is growing at around 6% a year[12]. Repeat prescriptions are a high proportion of the total: estimates vary between 70% and 80%. Almost all are generated by computer and printed at the GP practice, often by administrative staff for authorisation by the prescribing GP. Most of these are then collected by the patient, who, in the case of repeat prescriptions, will generally have to go to the practice for no other purpose than to pick up a paper script and carry it to the pharmacist. Around 30% of the paper scripts are collected, at patients' request, by pharmacies. The electronic transfer of prescriptions (ETP) from GP practice to pharmacy is intended, in part, to save everyone that little bit of bother. It will also make the process simpler in other ways. At the moment, information from the scripts has to be typed into computers at the pharmacy, where it forms part of the patient's medication record. Pharmacies subsequently forward the scripts to the prescription pricing authority (PPA), where information is again transcribed from the paper script to a computer system. If the scripts are electronic, all this information can be extracted automatically, saving time and reducing the risk of transcription errors. Enhanced communication between GP and pharmacy systems should also increase the information available at both ends and improve the quality of advice that both professions give to patients.

The promise, therefore, is considerable. Numerous reports, including the NHS Plan but also an Audit Commission report and a Chief Pharmaceutical Officer's report on medication errors, have highlighted the need for a greater role for IT in the prescribing process[13,14]. In 1998 the Department of Health published an information strategy with, among its goals, network connections between community pharmacies and GP practices by 2001[15]. A later paper, 'Pharmacy in the Future – Implementing the NHS plan' set a date of 2004 for the implementation of a nationwide system for the ETP[16]. Three pilot projects were commissioned, involving computer systems suppliers, pharmacies and NHS organisations. The pilot projects were all set up, run, evaluated and, in July 2003, discontinued. None of the piloted systems is to be made the basis for a more extensive roll-out of ETP. Such a roll-out is, however, planned as part of the National Programme for IT.

The evaluation of ETP

A report of the evaluation notes that many potential benefits were identified, but makes it clear that they were not, in fact, observed[17]. The take-up of ETP was much slower than expected, only achieving significant volumes at the end of the evaluation period (a total of 100 000 prescriptions had been anticipated; actually only 30 000 were generated). This was blamed in part on the fact that patients had to provide signed permission before their prescriptions could be transferred electronically and this proved a time-consuming process.

The lesson seems to be that although ETP looks like a good idea, the benefits are hard to achieve. One might have expected, for example, that if the prescription were sent in advance, patients would not have to spend so long waiting for medicines to be dispensed. Actually, difficulties staff had using the new systems meant that the reverse was true. And, if this was the case, the improved quality of service that was expected to follow from the freeing up of pharmacists' time could not have occurred. One of the most significant barriers to up-take was probably that the current system works relatively well for GPs. If the change is costly in terms of GP time, and the evidence is that it is, it is going to be hard to persuade GPs to make the changes that will save time for patients and pharmacists. One obvious way of saving GP time is removing the responsibility for the authorisation of repeat prescriptions, or at least automating the process by which such prescriptions are signed. Most GPs, however, were uncomfortable with this idea, and in two of the pilot projects a paper signature was created even for prescriptions that were transferred electronically, authorised under digital signature (see Box 14.1).

Looking at these pilot projects, together with evaluations of similar projects in the USA, the message seems to be that the expected benefits of ETP will be achieved, if at all, only after a period in which any benefit, in terms of time saved or quality of service improved, is outweighed by the costs involved in making the change. Mundy and Chadwick write that the prescription system is an 'irreversible' system, one that consists of highly entrenched actor-networks where complex interdependencies between the elements of the network make it particularly difficult to change[18]. They note that the only place where the anticipated efficiency benefits should be realised quickly and definitely is at the PPA; however, even there the likelihood is that the new system will have to run in parallel with the old system during the changeover period, which will substantially reduce the scope for savings.

Health informatics and ETP

The idea behind ETP seems deceptively simple. Instead of a patient having to collect a paper script and physically carry it to the pharmacy, it is sent electronically. We replace a simple physical act with an electronic one that should be comparably simple. Why is it, then, so difficult? Partly the reasons are to do with the social, clinical and legal processes that are involved in the creation and transmission of the paper document. Many people, notably many of the GPs in the pilot projects, are uncomfortable with the unfamiliar notion of a digital signature (see Box 14.1), and while recognising the potential benefits, they are anxious about the consequences of teething problems in the changeover. Others are aware that the existing processes allow for a certain level of flexibility and are worried that, particularly because one of the goals of ETP is to reduce fraud, its introduction might introduce awkward restrictions, for example, on procedures for modifying prescriptions.

Box 14.1 Dual key encryption

If you multiply together
9807508642406493739712550055038649119906436234252670840
6385189575946388957261768583317

and
4727721461074353025362230719730482246329146953020971164598527113052071125636359039 7527

you get:
188198812920607963838697239461650439807163563379417382700763356422988859715234665485319060606504743045317388011303396716199692321205734031879550656996221305168759307650257059.

You are probably prepared to trust me on this, but if you were not, you *could* check it: after all if you can do long multiplications, you can do very, very long multiplications. Imagine, however, the reverse problem. What if you were given the third number (call it *n*) and asked to find out which two numbers (call them *p* and *q*) were multiplied together to create it? There is not an easy way to do this. It is basically a matter of trial and error and the bigger the number, the longer it will take. A team in Germany devoted an enormous amount of energy to identifying the factors of *n*, a result they announced on 3 December 2003[1]. They took the trouble partly because a group called RSA Security was offering a $10 000 prize for the result, but partly, one suspects, for the fun of it.

RSA Security has an interest in such problems because they deal in encryption. The RSA algorithm is an example of what is known as dual key encryption. Before it was published in 1977, all known encryption algorithms relied on a single key shared by sender and receiver, so the basis for encrypting a message had to be agreed in advance and kept secret by both parties. The trick in dual key encryption is that there are two keys: a public one and a private one. How they are used depends on the application. The public key can be used to encrypt a message so that only the holder of the private key can decrypt it. This, obviously, is useful for sending confidential information across public networks. Alternatively the private key can be used to encrypt the message. Anyone with access to the public key can then decrypt the message. The message contents are not secure; the point is that if the decryption works, the message could only have come from the holder of the private key. This is the basis for approaches to authentication known as digital signatures, or digital certificates.

(*continued*)

Box 14.1 Dual key encryption (*continued*)

The two keys have to be linked, but a neat piece of mathematics means that it can be made very hard – as hard as finding p and q given n – to work out the private key from the public key. The RSA algorithm works as follows: take two large primes, p and q, and compute their product $n = pq$. Choose a number, e, less than n such that e and $(p-1)(q-1)$ have no common factors. Find another number d such that $(ed - 1)$ is divisible by $(p-1)$ and $(q-1)$. Another way of saying that $(ed-1)$ is divisible by $(p-1)$ would be to say that if ed is divided by $(p-1)$, the remainder is 1, or that ed and 1 are congruent, modulo $(p-1)$. We can write this constraint, and that for $(q-1)$, using the notation for modular arithmetic:

$$ed \equiv 1 (\text{mod } p - 1) \text{ and } ed \equiv 1 (\text{mod } q - 1) \qquad (1)$$

The public key is the pair (n, e); the private key is (n, d).

Before we can use RSA, the message must first be turned into a number, perhaps by concatenating ASCII codes for the alphanumeric characters in the message. Imagine we want to encrypt a message m so that only the recipient can decrypt it. To encrypt m, we obtain the recipient's public key (n, e) and calculate the remainder when m is raised to the power e and the result divided by n:

$$c = m^e \text{mod } n \qquad (2)$$

The remainder c is the encrypted message. To decrypt c, the recipient uses his or her private key (n, d) to calculate:

$$m = c^d \text{mod } n$$

It might not be immediately apparent why this should work, how can d reverse a process that used e? And what has n got to do with it? The answer lies in an elegant theorem known as Fermat's little theorem: for any integer a and any prime p, $a^p \equiv a (\text{mod } p)$. That is to say, if you raise a to the power p and then divide the result by p, the remainder is a. A generalisation of the theorem states that if p is prime and m and n are integers such that $m \equiv n (\text{mod } p - 1)$, then $a^m \equiv a^n (\text{mod } p)$ for any a. The magic of RSA happens in the application of this generalisation to the definition of d in (1). This gives:

$$m^{ed} \equiv m (\text{mod } p) \text{ and } m^{ed} \equiv m (\text{mod } q)$$

from which it follows, although not quite straightforwardly, that:

$$m^{ed} \equiv m (\text{mod } n)$$

and hence, readily, from (2):

(*continued*)

> **Box 14.1 Dual key encryption** (*continued*)
>
> $c^d \equiv m(\bmod n)$
>
> It is worth noting that the choice of number for d, the private exponent, is constrained by the values of e, p and q. The values of e and n are public. So if anyone were to find an easy way of working out p and q, given n, it would not be too hard to find d, and RSA would no longer be secure. In the mean time, the prize helps RSA Security judge just how hard it is to factor the product of two very large prime numbers. Every time someone factors the RSA challenge number, the company knows that primes used to create n have to be made even larger. At the time of writing a $20 000 prize is being offered for the factors of:
> 3107418240490004372135075003588856793003734602284272754572016194882320644051808150455634682967172328678243791627283803341547107310850191954852900733772482278352574238645401469173660247765234660$9^2$.
>
> 1. http://www.rsasecurity.com/ rsalabs/node.asp?id=2096
> 2. http://www.rsasecurity.com/ rsalabs/node.asp?id=2214

There are, however, some technical issues that need to be addressed. The aim, actually, is not simply to replace the physical transfer of a script with an electronic transfer. The aim is also to automate the process by which the information on the script is inserted into the computer systems at the pharmacy and at the PPA. There is, therefore, a requirement for a common terminology to be used in the various systems. At first glance, it would seem easier to agree on a standard set of terms here than in various clinical domains tackled in Chapter 9; however, there are still problems because the terminology used in prescribing is different from that used in dispensing. The clinician wants to be able to prescribe a drug at a defined dose, and the pharmacist needs to identify a package on the shelf. Essentially what is required are two terminology standards: one for the clinician and another for the pharmacist, and a mapping between the two.

Standards for electronic prescribing

In the USA, the National Council for Prescription Drug Programs has published the *NCPDP* script standard to facilitate the electronic transmission of information between clinicians and pharmacists[19]. It is a messaging standard, supporting a defined number of transactions: new prescription, prescription change request, refill prescription, cancel prescription, etc. Each message contains a set of segments: header, clinician segment, pharmacist segment, patient segment and drug segment. The first four contain the kind of information you would expect: for example, the pharmacist segment contains a standard ID number, name, address, etc.; the drug segment contains a mix of text strings (indicating drug name, strength and form, and also the patient

directions, e.g. 'one tablet by mouth three times a day') and standard iden-
tifiers. It is left to implementers to choose whether to transfer 'Amoxicillin|
chewable tablet|500 mg|by mouth|three times a day' or 'NDC 1234567890
po tid'. The latter is a code that is useful in pharmacy systems, distinguishing
between brands, subforms and packages of the same drug, but which is far too
specific to be of value in clinical systems.

The NHS Information Authority has published a dictionary of medicines
and devices (dm+d)[20]. The dictionary is based on a model that distinguishes
between the kinds of thing a clinician would prescribe and the kinds of thing
a pharmacist would dispense. The core concepts in the model are:

- 'Virtual therapeutic moiety' – the abstract representation of the substance,
  formulated as a medicinal product, that a prescriber might intend for use in
  treating a patient, e.g. paracetamol.
- 'Virtual medicinal product' – an abstract concept capturing one or more
  actual medicinal products, e.g. 1% hydrocortisone cream.
- 'Actual medicinal product' – a single dose unit of a finished dose form, e.g.
  atenolol 100 mg tablets (Alpharma).
- 'Virtual medicinal product pack' – an abstract concept representing one or
  more equivalent actual medicinal product packs, e.g. generic Estracombi
  TTS patches × 8 patches.
- 'Actual medicinal product pack' – the packaged product supplied direct for
  patient use, e.g. 28 tablets of AstraZeneca Tenormin 100 mg tablets.

Each concept is defined, in the familiar UML terminology, through associations with other concepts, and each has a set of attributes, including, where
appropriate, a reference to a SNOMED CT identifier.

ETP and decision support

The computerisaton of prescribing might seem a good idea because of the scope
that it allows for decision support, which in turn would allow for automated
checking for known allergies and drug–drug interactions. It should be remembered, however, that computerised decision support for prescribing is really a
separate issue from the electronic *transmission* of prescriptions. The provision of
decision support to the prescriber is no simpler because the prescription is sent
electronically from the prescriber's computer than it was when the prescription was printed out on paper. Improved communication between the prescribing GP and the dispensing pharmacist might allow for improved decision
support but that seems unlikely to change the existing situation. The fact that
the prescriptions arrive from the GP's surgery electronically might reduce the
scope for error at the pharmacy, but achieving that gain depends on how the
new technology is incorporated into the dispensing process.

Conclusion

At the time of writing it is unclear whether Connecting for Health will
be viewed as a success. Significant progress has been made on both the

Choose and Book and the ETP programmes but much remains to be done. Success will be a matter not just of good design and engineering but also of organisational change and straightforward politics. Among the aims of health informatics researchers is the development of standards and other tools that could help solve some of the problems, but only some. Health informatics, however, is a field with broader horizons and longer-term goals than those of Connecting for Health. Chapter 15, the final chapter, reflects on some of these and on key topics identified in the course of the book.

References

1. Iles V, Sutherland K. *Organisational Change: A Review for Health Care Managers, Professionals and Researchers*. London: National Co-ordinating Centre for Service Delivery and Organisation, 2002.
2. Department of Health. *The NHS Plan: A Plan for Investment, a Plan for Reform*. London: HMSO, 2000.
3. Berwick DM. A primer on leading the improvement of systems. *BMJ* 1996;312(7031):619–622.
4. Kerr D, Bevan H, Gowland B, Penny J, Berwick D. Redesigning cancer care. *BMJ* 2002;324(7330):164–166.
5. Garvey CJ, Seymour R, Wright L. Radiology and the Cancer Services Collaborative – an opportunity awaits. *Clin Radiol* 2003;58(2):97–101. Review.
6. Ham C, Kipling R, McLeod H. Redesigning work processes in health care: lessons from the National Health Service. *Milbank Q* 2003;81(3):415–439.
7. McLeod H, Ham C, Kipling R. Booking patients for hospital admissions: evaluation of a pilot programme for day cases. *BMJ* 2003;327(7424):1147.
8. Utley M, Gallivan S, Treasure T, Valencia O. Analytical methods for calculating the capacity required to operate an effective booked admissions policy for elective inpatient services. *Health Care Manag Sci* 2003;6(2):97–104.
9. Gallivan S, Utley M, Treasure T, Valencia O. Booked inpatient admissions and hospital capacity: mathematical modelling study. *BMJ* 2002;324(7332):280–282.
10. McKusker S, Holcroft T, Hackett, P. Electronic booking and directories of service: a systematic approach to development. *Br J Healthcare Comput Inf Manag* 2004;21(6):21–26.
11. Electronic Prescribing Initiative. *Electronic Prescribing: Toward Maximum Value and Rapid Adoption*. Washington, DC: eHealth Initiative, 2004.
12. NHS National Programme for IT. *Electronic Transmission of Prescriptions*. NHS Executive, 2004. http://www.npfit.nhs.uk/programmes/etp
13. Audit Commission. *A Spoonful of Sugar: Medicines Management in NHS Hospitals*. London: Audit Commission, 2001.
14. Chief Pharmaceutical Officer. *Building a Safer NHS for Patients: Improving Medication Safety*. London: Department of Health, 2004.
15. Department of Health. *Information for Health*. London: Department of Health, 1999.
16. Department of Health. *Pharmacy in the Future: Implementing the NHS Plan*. Department of Health, 2004.

17. Sugden R. *Electronic Transmission of Prescriptions Evaluation of Pilots: Summary Report.* Sowerby Centre for Health Informatics at Newcastle, 2004.
18. Mundy D, Chadwick DW. Electronic transmission of prescriptions: towards realizing the dream. *Int J Electronic Healthcare* 2004;1(1):112–125.
19. The National Council for Prescription Drug Programmes. *The National Council for Prescription Drug Programmes.* http://www.ncpdp.org/main_frame.htm (accessed on 24 May 2005).
20. The UK Standard Clinical Products Reference Source Programme (UKCPRSP). *NHS Dictionary of Medicines and Devices Technical Specification Release 2.* London: NHS Information Authority, 2004.

CHAPTER 15
Conclusions

This book presents a brief survey of health informatics. Its organising theme is a virtuous cycle in which the improved collection of patient data leads to advances in medical knowledge that are then translated into better outcomes for new patients, whose data is collected in turn and analysed to allow further advances. Although the book focuses on the collection, management and analysis of data, and on tools that give practitioners better access to clinical evidence and medical knowledge, there is other work that also deserves to be mentioned. Before reviewing the main themes of the book I want, in this concluding chapter, to give some pointers to two other areas of health informatics research: consumer health informatics and health technology.

Consumer health informatics

Most of the work described in this book was done to support clinical work, to help health professionals deliver care. Increasingly, however, researchers are considering how health informatics can be applied to help patients look after themselves. Very often when we are ill, or even when we are quite well but thinking and making decisions about our health, we do so without directly involving a health professional. There are good reasons why it is worth encouraging people to look after themselves; it reduces pressure on professionals and can also enhance patients' sense of control over their condition.

There are a variety of ways in which health informatics can help patients as well as doctors. The following subsections deal with five of these ways: health information websites, patient access to records, decision support tools, interactive health care applications and Internet support groups.

Health information websites

As well as giving clinicians access to the best available medical knowledge, the Internet can also be used to help patients find information about their conditions and treatments. There are many examples of such websites, including the *BMJ Best Treatment Guide to Clinical Evidence*[1]. The issues involved in designing information sources for patients are very different from those in designing tools for clinicians. A clinician has to deal with large numbers of patients, all with different problems, and can spend only a little time searching for the answer to a question. The situation is reversed for a patient whose interests are much more focused, and who can invest more time in researching a question. In some ways, therefore, designing information sources for patients is easier than designing them for clinicians. Clinicians, however, are able to draw on a great deal of useful background knowledge in searching for information. As experts they know where to look for new information, and how to assess its quality.

It is extremely easy to publish information on the Web and once information is published, it is available to everyone with access to the Internet. One of the concerns of researchers looking at consumer health information on the Internet has been how to control the quality of information provided. In one study of consumer health information a breast oncologist reviewed a sample of pages from the first 200 websites returned when entering the term 'breast cancer' into Google[2]. The sample contained 184 sites with information about breast cancer, 12 of which contained inaccurate medical statements.

There have been at least 13 different initiatives to develop quality and ethical standards for health information on the Internet[3]. For example, the Health on the Net (HON) Foundation, a non-profit organisation established in 1995, and funded primarily by Swiss governmental organisations, proposes the HONcode, which sets out eight ethical principles, shown in Table 15.1, for health information websites[4]. Sites that conform to these principles are allowed to display the HONcode logo on their pages. Risk and Dzenowagis argue that any successful quality initiative would require not just a set of quality criteria but also a credible enforcement initiative[3]: the Meric et al. review of breast cancer websites, mentioned above, found that some sites displaying the HON logo did not comply with the HONcode[2].

Recently researchers have begun to worry less about the fact that there is poor quality information on the Web and to look more carefully at how the public search for, and make use of, health information. One observational study, for example, investigated how patients assess the credibility of a site[5]. A variety of criteria seem to be used, with professional design being more significant than the credibility of the organisation responsible for the site. In fact users seem rarely to check who is responsible for a site and typically forget from which site they retrieved information. Users generally carry out multiple searches and look, albeit briefly, at a number of different sites in attempting to answer a question. The authors concluded that where consumers arrived at the wrong answer having used the Internet, it was because they had misunderstood information and not because they had been misinformed.

Patient access to records

One of the consequences of moving from a paper-based record to an electronic record is that it becomes easier to share patient data between different physicians. There are also potential benefits in allowing patients access to their records. Patients in many countries already have the right to see their records. Having a right of access, however, is not the same as having access,

Table 15.1 The HONcode for health information on the Internet.

1 Authority
Any medical or health advice provided and hosted on this site will only be given by medically trained and qualified professionals unless a clear statement is made that a piece of advice offered is from a non-medically qualified individual or organisation.

2 Complementarity
The information provided on this site is designed to support, not replace, the relationship that exists between a patient / site visitor and his/her existing physician.

3 Confidentiality
Confidentiality of data relating to individual patients and visitors to a medical/health website, including their identity, is respected by this website. The website owners undertake to honour or exceed the legal requirements of medical/health information privacy that apply in the country and state where the website and mirror sites are located.

4 Attribution
Where appropriate, information contained on this site will be supported by clear references to source data and, where possible, have specific HTML links to that data. The date when a clinical page was last modified will be clearly displayed.

5 Justifiability
Any claims relating to the benefits/performance of a specific treatment, commercial product or service will be supported by appropriate, balanced evidence in the manner outlined above in Principle 4.

6 Transparency of authorship
The designers of this website will seek to provide information in the clearest possible manner and provide contact addresses for visitors who seek further information or support. The Webmaster will display his/her email address clearly throughout the website.

7 Transparency of sponsorship
Support for this website will be clearly identified, including the identities of commercial and non-commercial organisations that have contributed funding, services or material for the site.

8 Honesty in advertising and editorial policy
If advertising is a source of funding, it will be clearly stated. A brief description of the advertising policy adopted by the website owners will be displayed on the site. Advertising and other promotional material will be presented to viewers in a manner and context that facilitates differentiation between it and the original material created by the institution operating the site.

and in practice it is relatively rare that patients ask to see their records. One of the proposals under the current UK National Programme for IT is the creation of 'My HealthSpace' through which patients will be able to access their records via the Web[6]. What might this mean?

A recent review of pilot studies in which patients were given the opportunity to view their records found evidence of modest improvements in doctor–patient communication, adherence to medication, patient empowerment and patient education[7]. There is also evidence that some patients find parts of their record difficult to understand. For a few patients the experience of seeing their record is confusing or upsetting. The benefits seem to outweigh the problems, however. There are serious issues that still need to be resolved: for example, the problem of patients discovering 'bad news' before a planned doctor–patient consultation or the risk of losing third-party confidentiality.

The review found many instances where patients identified errors in the record. One study found 68% of psychiatric patients reported that access to the record allowed them to correct inaccurate information[8]. This raises an interesting point. It is generally assumed that access is read-only. But why should patients not alter their records? One of the innovative aspects of My HealthSpace is that patients will also be able to record information, for example, noting their use of 'over the counter' medicines or complementary therapies. Mandl *et al.* have argued that patients should be given not just access to but also control over their records[9]. They should, it is proposed, be able to decide who should have access to their data, how it should be used and also be allowed to annotate and modify the record. Perhaps unsurprisingly while patients tend to support the idea of access, physicians have more concerns and perceive less potential benefit. Winning physicians over to the idea that patients should have not just access but control may take some time.

Decision support tools

Tools, such as those described in Chapter 10, that help to elicit patients' preferences for different possible outcomes and decide on an appropriate course of action in the light of those preferences inevitably involve the patient in taking a more active role in the decision. In theory there is no reason why computerised decision support tools should only be designed for settings where a clinician is guiding the patient. In some situations, it might well be more appropriate to make the tool available to the patient so that he or she can use it by himself or herself. For example, Barratt *et al.* describe a tool designed to help women weigh up the pros and cons of breast cancer screening[10]. They suggest that the tool could be used by clinicians to help patients make a choice consistent with their own circumstances and preferences. However, most women will make this decision without consulting a health professional, and it is clearly possible to make a version of the tool available via the Web for women to consult directly.

Schwitzer identified five consumer decision support tools, only one of which presented information tailored to the individual[11]. The NexCura Cancer Profiler™ elicits information about the user's diagnosis and test results, matches it with information about research studies and gives advice on treatment options and outcomes. At present there are relatively few such tools but it seems likely that they will become more common.

Interactive health care applications

Interactive websites can solicit personal details from users and present tailored information that reflects the users' circumstances. Such interactive applications have been developed for health care, on CD-ROMs as well as on websites. Some are intended not just to provide information or support decision-making but also to have a therapeutic effect. Systems have been developed for various forms of cognitive behavioural therapy, to help with depression, insomnia, headache, problem drinking and smoking cessation[12–16].

For example, Clarke et al. have carried out a number of studies of a program designed to deliver a form of cognitive behavioural therapy that assists patients with depression[12]. Unusually this intervention, which is delivered via the Internet, is 'pure self-help': there is no therapist involved. The patient interacts with the website and thereby acquires skills that help modify behaviour and improve well-being. In trials of these kinds of systems 'guided self-help', in which there is limited access to a therapist as well as some form of computer-based interactive tool, has been found effective, but pure self-help systems have had little or no impact. Clarke et al. note that in their early studies it was clear that participants randomised to pure self-help tended to stop using the site fairly quickly. In this study they incorporated a system of reminders (either letters or short telephone calls) and found that the impact of the site was significantly improved.

The idea of using an interactive tool to deliver a health care intervention is not new. Indeed one of the earliest attempts at artificial intelligence involved a program called Eliza, which carried out simplistic syntactic analysis of typed input in order to generate a meaningful reply that would serve to solicit further input[17]. The aim was to encourage the user to keep typing, exactly as a Rogerian therapist encourages patients to keep talking and so reveal their concerns.

Internet support groups

One of the difficulties with interactive health care applications is the lack of a human dimension to the intervention. The Internet is, however, as much a social as a technical phenomenon and many patients have found that they can use it not just to access information but also to contact other patients with similar conditions and in similar situations.

Internet support groups represent a form of health care innovation in which health care professionals play almost no role. They have, however, been studied in order to assess their impact. Lorig et al. describe a trial in which patients with back pain were randomly assigned to either an email discussion list or usual care[18]. After a year the intervention group were found to have improved health status and to have made fewer visits to their physician.

A review of research in the field identified ten studies of Internet support groups for cancer patients and noted that six of them dealt with breast cancer[19]. The potential benefit of Internet support groups is, however, perhaps greatest for rare conditions, for which it would not be possible to create a conventional face-to-face support group. Lasker *et al.* analysed the content of messages posted to a mailing list for patients with a rare disease: primary biliary cirrhosis[20]. They concluded that the Internet provided a highly valued outlet, particularly for those who are newly diagnosed and in need of health information, but that it is an important resource for people at all stages of the disease.

Health technology

One of the challenges in understanding how to apply IT to the problems of health care is in keeping pace with progress in the development of the underlying technology. For most of this book the focus has been on information and on software that deals with information; in this section it is on the technology, on the hardware.

Robots

The most obviously high-tech form of medical hardware is perhaps the surgical robot. Commercial robots have been around for about 40 years and have been widely used in industry since the 1970s. They excel at tasks that are repeatable and that require precision. Although surgery requires precision, each patient is different, meaning that robots cannot be pre-programmed to carry out an operation in the way they can be programmed to assemble a car.

Surgical robots now exist for a variety of tasks, carried out with varying degrees of input from the surgeon. Some robots provide the surgeon with enhanced access and improved control. For example, to avoid damaging retinal blood vessels – and inadvertently blinding the patient – an ophthalmic surgeon must position his or her laser within 25 μm of the target. Unaided, the human hand cannot reliably direct a surgical instrument to within less than 100 μm. To make matters worse the natural motion of the eye means the target will be moving. Using computer-assisted surgical tools, the motion of the eye can be tracked and the surgeon's tremor can be filtered, allowing the laser to be positioned within 10 μm of a target[21]. Other systems, which are integrated with imaging systems, operate more or less autonomously while the procedure is executed. One example would be the CyberKnife linear accelerator[22]. The accelerator is used in conjunction with CT and MRI images taken before the treatment starts. The images are registered with images taken during the procedure and the results used to control the robotic arm on which the accelerator is mounted, so that it can adjust, in real time, to movements in the target, meaning that the patient no longer needs to be immobilised.

The next generation of surgical robots is expected to take this integration of imaging and navigation a step further. Significant progress is also expected in the miniaturisation of robots. Existing systems augment the performance of surgeons tackling the kind of procedures that can otherwise be done manually. Rapidly advancing research in micro-electrical mechanical systems means that surgeons will soon be able to contemplate surgical manipulations on the micro-scale, carrying out procedures that are completely different to those performed today.

Miniaturisation could extend beyond the micro- to the nano-scale, at which point it is possible to consider robots that could fit inside a single living cell or travel around the body in the bloodstream. One application of such nanotechnology would be in the treatment of diabetes: a single implantable device could not just measure glucose levels continuously but also respond to the measurements and deliver insulin as needed[23].

Telemonitoring

The management of diabetes is already being influenced by the availability of portable, although by no means nano-scale, glucose meters. The self-monitoring of diabetes is now common practice[24]. Patients with hypertension are increasingly being given access to blood pressure monitors at home[25]. Other 'telemonitoring' initiatives have dealt with problems such as heart failure[26].

Cappuccio *et al.* reviewed the research on home monitoring of blood pressure and found that patients monitoring their blood pressure at home had better control and were more likely to achieve targets[25].

The real promise of this kind of telemonitoring technology is that it allows patients to become self-managing. There is therefore a strong connection between this research and consumer health informatics. Self-management involves not just being able to measure one's glucose level or blood pressure but also being able to make an appropriate response to the measurement. Kelham argues that informed self-regulation is the next step and cites successful small-scale studies of self-medication in hypertension and anticoagulation[27]. In a different study, asthmatic patients who adjusted their drug treatment using a written plan ended up with improved lung function compared to those whose treatment was adjusted by a doctor[28].

Telemedicine

Telemonitoring is just one approach to what is known as telemedicine, the use of information and communication technology to overcome barriers associated with distance in the practice of medicine. A nineteenth-century physician dispatching a letter of advice, or a doctor 50 years ago discussing a case over the telephone, would have been practising medicine at a distance. It was, however, only at the end of the 1960s, when the use of television allowed a doctor to see and hear a patient at a distant location, that a very few people began to talk of 'telemedicine'. In the 1990s, the term became rather fashionable and a plethora of journals and conferences about telemedicine appeared. Now, however, fashion seems to be moving on.

The availability of cheap computer power and high-bandwidth telecommunications networks has made the rapid transfer of digital data part of everyday life. The term 'telemedicine' exists because computer-derived images transmitted over digital networks have made us think about how medicine might be practised at a distance. But even if it is technology that has raised the question, it does not follow that technology is, necessarily, the solution. We have to focus on the underlying issue of how the players (patients, GPs, specialists) in health care can communicate more effectively, using the range of technological options open to them. A 1997 review of 80 trials of 'electronic communication' with patients found many successful examples of innovative uses of relatively low-tech telephone services in counselling, reminders, follow-up and other applications – including consultation services analogous to NHSdirect[29].

In contrast, although videoconferencing has become an established tool for delivering health care in settings where there are sparse populations and real geographical difficulties, attempts to demonstrate its effectiveness in urban settings, for example, as a means of improving communication between primary and secondary care in the UK, have largely failed. In one case, patients being referred by their GP were randomly assigned to either a conventional outpatient appointment or to a 'virtual outreach' appointment, in which the patient would return to the GP surgery for a videoconference with the consultant[30]. The trial found that patients liked the service but that consultants were reluctant to rely on the GP's examination, with the consequence that an additional outpatient appointment was often generated.

Although telemedicine seems to be a less fashionable area of research now than it was perhaps 10 years ago, there is still some merit in looking at certain problems in health informatics as communication problems, the solutions for which will be the design of appropriate communication channels. Traditionally health informatics has focused, as indeed this book has, on systems to help clinicians manage patient data, process information and access knowledge; the development of systems to support effective communication is a relatively new approach.

Grids

When you look at a Web page, what you see on your screen is the result of downloading HTML files from another computer. The great thing about the Web is that you can look at pages without needing to know anything about the computer on which they are stored. Imagine a network whose users shared not just HTML files but all sorts of software, data and processing power. Just as your Web browser conceals all the work involved in retrieving files across a network, a different but equally straightforward interface could execute programs, run database queries and analyse data on any networked computer and you would see the results without needing to know which machines performed the operations. Such networks are called grids. The term was originally applied to what are now called computational grids: virtual supercomputers in which the processing power of a large number of machines is aggregated to tackle complex problems. Other forms of grid have been proposed: knowledge grids – rather like the Semantic Web – that support knowledge sharing and reuse; and collaborative grids that support distributed cooperative work.

Grids, in fact, do not require special hardware. The development of grids requires special software, known as middleware, to allow the networked computers to be treated as a grid. Grid technology is being applied to the most computationally intractable and data-intensive tasks facing science. Many of these problems are in biomedicine and grids are being developed to deal with them. Examples being considered include the processing of large numbers of medical images, the execution of simulations modelling complex processes, large-scale epidemiological studies and data mining in pharmaceutical research[31].

Clinical work and technological change

The early years of the twenty-first century have seen a shift in the relationship between patients and health professionals, as the former grow more knowledgeable and more assertive. As the research surveyed above illustrates, patients have increasing access not just to better information about health care but also to software applications and, in some cases, medical devices that allow them to play an increasingly active role in monitoring and managing their health. These changes are, of course, not universal: not all clinical roles are affected, not all patients seek to be more involved in clinical decisions.

IT changes clinical roles in other ways. Many specialities, such as surgery and radiology, require clinicians to master increasingly complex and specialised tools, and to do so with greater frequency. The discipline of health informatics is, in part, an agent of technological change, creating new tools and requiring clinicians to adapt to them. It is, however, in part an approach to dealing with such change. Research in health informatics aims to understand what is essential about clinical work and to design appropriate tools. Good design, which includes effective techniques for understanding how clinical work is carried out and eliciting the requirements for effective clinical systems, is a crucial element here.

The rest of this chapter returns to the theme of this book – how the effective management of patient data can be used to improve care – and considers the prospects for future work.

The principles and practice of health informatics

Chapter 6 dealt with logic. It might have seemed strange to some readers to be going back to a field of enquiry that dates back to Aristotle. It certainly seems a long step from propositional calculus to the kinds of projects described in Chapter 14, the electronic transfer of prescriptions (ETP), for example. The significance of logic to health informatics is that it enables computations (inferences) to be carried out on abstract representations of knowledge (sets of propositions). Such representations might be termed 'logical models'. They include the ontologies described in Chapters 8 and 9 for supporting SNOMED CT and other controlled clinical terminologies, standards such as HL7 and projects such as openEHR. The ETP project employs a standard terminology for pharmaceutical products, the dm+d. The development of such a standard involves building the kinds of abstract models logic deals with. Incorporating decision support into ETP requires the representation of clinical knowledge in the form of logical rules for safe prescribing. The development and application of such models is the core business of health informatics.

From patient data to medical knowledge

Developing tools to support the three grand challenges identified in Part 1 involves applying these modelling techniques to a range of problems. Building systems to support the first challenge – improving the recording and management of patient data – involves working with controlled clinical terminologies to ensure that information is recorded consistently. This is important if data are to be aggregated for audit, or to support management. It is also important if the data are to be shared, for example, between primary and secondary care providers. The sharing of patient data can also require the use of messaging standards such as HL7. The next section describes a project in which data recorded using a controlled clinical terminology are analysed to tackle the second grand challenge – using patient data to extend medical knowledge.

General practice research database

In the late 1980s, a number of companies were set up to sell various forms of IT solution to general practitioners. One, VAMP Health, had a particularly attractive business model in that GPs were provided with free software and hardware on the condition that they provide VAMP with data about morbidity, drug prescribing and side-effects. VAMP hoped to make a profit by selling the data to the pharmaceutical industry but in 1993 ownership passed to Reuters Health Care who donated the database to the Department of Health[32]. The General Practice Research Database (GPRD), as it is now known, is administered by the UK Medicines and Health Care products Regulatory Agency (MHRA) and is now the largest and most comprehensive database of its kind, containing records from a total of 9 million patients, from almost 400 primary care practices[33]. Over 400 publications have reported research carried out using the database.

By way of an example of the kind of research that can be conducted with the database, take a recent paper from a well-known journal. Cleary *et al.* carried out a study in which 4709 individuals with idiopathic epilepsy beginning after the age of 60 years were identified from the GPRD, and 4709 matching controls were selected, in order to test the hypothesis that late onset epileptic seizures is a predictor of stroke[34]. The authors report that there were 471 strokes among patients in the study cohort (10.0%) compared to 207 in the control group (4.4%), an absolute difference of 5.6% (95% CI 4.6–6.7). The study provides pretty striking evidence of an effect and suggests that a patient who first has seizures late in life is at increased risk of stroke and, the authors argue, should be screened for vascular risk factors and treated appropriately.

This kind of retrospective review is considered methodologically inferior to prospective trial, since the data were not collected specifically in order to answer this question. There might, for example, be a bias whereby the data on patients who had had seizures were more complete than that for the controls (although in this case the experimenters offer some guarantees that this was not so). However, the increasingly restrictive regulatory framework for clinical research means that the use of archive data is highly appealing.

There is a limit on the kind of research that can be done with the GPRD, because there is a limit on the amount of data that is recorded for the patients it contains. There is a great deal of valuable detail about prescriptions, referrals, immunisations, tests results and some lifestyle information. Free text information is also available. In practice, however, most research will be done using the coded data about the patients' diagnoses, symptoms, procedures and medical history, and therefore can only be analysed at the level of detail at which GPs record information using clinical codes.

CLEF

Another approach to creating an archive of clinical data for research purposes involves the analysis of free text. Progress in programming computers to understand 'natural' language has been much slower than the early pioneers of artificial intelligence anticipated. There has, however, been progress, and within circumscribed domains computers can be used to identify concepts from passages of free text. Some researchers are now applying this technology to analyse patient histories and reports in order to extract the kind of information that clinicians have not, up to now, recorded using clinical codes. The Clinical eScience Framework (CLEF) is using grid technology to create an archive of patient data that can be used to answer research questions[35].

A key difference between CLEF and the GPRD is that CLEF uses natural language processing technology to extract key concepts from narrative entries in the patient record. This is held to be tractable in part because CLEF deals only with cancer patients and therefore has to handle only a very limited range of language, dealing with a well-defined list of possible events. Another important point is that most events are described by multiple reports, which helps enormously in the resolution of ambiguities. The aim of CLEF's natural language processing is to assemble a chronicle that is drawn in part from the structured data items on the record, in part from the analysis of free text and in part from inferences drawn from this information. The set of patient chronicles will, it is hoped, allow researchers to answer significant questions about cancer and the effectiveness of cancer treatments.

Automated information extraction

If natural language processing can be made to work, and if it is being applied not just in CLEF but in a range of projects, then we can expect to see a dramatic shift in the scope and ambition of health informatics. A whole set of applications will become possible, including some that address the third of our grand challenges. Just as it will become possible to derive new knowledge from the information currently concealed in unanalysed text, it will become possible to answer queries by extracting existing knowledge from conventional texts. Already projects are attempting to use specialised knowledge of molecular biology to allow the automated analysis of scientific knowledge[36]. It is hard to assess the likely impact of this research, and given the history of the field a conservative estimate is probably prudent but it is one area where the dramatic changes that the IT industry has seen over the last 10 years – huge increases in the amount both of accessible electronic text and of computational power with which to process it – might make a real difference.

Conclusion

Presenting the aims of health informatics as a set of grand challenges might seem to suggest that these were problems for which a researcher might find a solution. That probably is not the appropriate way of looking at them. Each of the many different projects mentioned in this book is an attempt to solve part of the problem, to make a piecemeal improvement that will contribute to a process by which the delivery of health care is improved through the more intelligent use of IT and the more effective management of information.

Achieving these improvements will, in practice, require more than just successful academic research. The literature reviewed in Chapters 12–14 addresses some of the difficulties associated with organisational change. One reason for writing this book is that if these difficulties are to be overcome, health care professionals must acquire a greater understanding of health informatics, if they are to help improve the organisation and practice of health care in a technologically advanced and information-rich society.

References

1. BMJ Publishing Group. *Welcome to BestTreatments*. http://www.besttreatments. co.uk/btuk/home.html (accessed on 6 July 2005).
2. Meric F, Bernstam EV, Mirza NQ, Hunt KK, Ames FC, Ross MI, Kuerer HM, Pollock RE, Musen MA, Singletary SE. Breast cancer on the World Wide Web: cross-sectional survey of quality of information and popularity of websites. *BMJ* 2002;324(7337):577–581.
3. Risk A, Dzenowagis J. Review of Internet health information quality initiatives. *J Med Internet Res* 2001;3(4):E28.
4. Health on the Net Foundation HON Code of Conduct (HONcode) for medical and health web sites. http://www.hon.ch/HONcode/Conduct.html (accessed on 13 July 2005).
5. Eysenbach G, Kohler C. How do consumers search for and appraise health information on the World Wide Web? Qualitative study using focus groups, usability tests, and in-depth interviews. *BMJ* 2002;324(7337):573–577.
6. NHS Welcome to HealthSpace. http://www.healthspace.nhs.uk (accessed on 14 July 2005).
7. Ross SE, Lin CT. The effects of promoting patient access to medical records: a review. *J Am Med Inform Assoc* 2003;10(2):129–138.
8. Ross SE, Todd J, Moore LA, Beaty BL, Wittevrongel L, Lin CT. Expectations of patients and physicians regarding patient-accessible medical records. *J Med Internet Res* 2005;7(2):e13.
9. Mandl KD, Szolovits P, Kohane IS. Public standards and patients' control: how to keep electronic medical records accessible but private. *BMJ* 2001;322(7281):283–287.
10. Barratt A, Howard K, Irwig L, Salkeld G, Houssami N. Model of outcomes of screening mammography: information to support informed choices. *BMJ*;10.1136/ bmj.38398.469479.8F.
11. Schwitzer G. A review of features in Internet consumer health decision-support tools. *J Med Internet Res* 2002;4(2):E11.
12. Clarke G, Eubanks D, Reid E, Kelleher C, O'Connor E, DeBar L, Lynch F, Nunley S, Gullion C. Overcoming depression on the Internet (ODIN) (2): a randomized trial of a self-help depression Skills Program With Reminders. *J Med Internet Res* 2005;7(2): E16.
13. Strom L, Pettersson R, Andersson G. Internet-based treatment for insomnia: a controlled evaluation. *J Consult Clin Psychol* 2004;72(1):113–120.
14. Andersson G, Lundstrom P, Strom L. Internet-based treatment of headache: does telephone contact add anything? *Headache* 2003;43(4):353–361.
15. Kypri K, Saunders JB, Williams SM, McGee RO, Langley JD, Cashell-Smith ML, Gallagher SJ. Web-based screening and brief intervention for hazardous drinking: a double-blind randomized controlled trial. *Addiction* 2004;99(11):1410–1417.
16. Escoffery C, McCormick L, Bateman K. Development and process evaluation of a Web-based smoking cessation program for college smokers: innovative tool for education. *Patient Educ Couns* 2004;53(2):217–225.
17. Wikipedia Eliza. http://en.wikipedia.org/wiki/Eliza (accessed on 13 July 2005).
18. Lorig KR, Laurent DD, Deyo RA, Marnell ME, Minor MA, Ritter PL. Can a Back Pain E-mail Discussion Group improve health status and lower health care costs? A randomized study. *Arch Intern Med* 2002;162(7):792–796.

19. Klemm P, Bunnell D, Cullen M, Soneji R, Gibbons P, Holecek A. Online cancer support groups: a review of the research literature. *Comput Inform Nurs* 2003;21(3): 136–142.

20. Lasker J, Sogolow E, Sharim R. The role of an online community for people with a rare disease: content analysis of messages posted on a primary biliary cirrhosis mailing list. *J Med Internet Res* 2005;7(1):E12.

21. Camarillo DB, Krummel TM, Salisbury JK Jr. Robotic technology in surgery: past, present, and future. *Am J Surg* 2004;188(4A Suppl):2S–15S.

22. Mehta VK, Lee QT, Chang SD, Cherney S, Adler JR Jr. Image-guided stereotactic radiosurgery for lesions in proximity to the anterior visual pathways: a preliminary report. *Technol Cancer Res Treat* 2002;1(3):173–180.

23. Lanfranco AR, Castellanos AE, Desai JP, Meyers WC. Robotic surgery – a current perspective. *Ann Surg* 2004;239:14–21.

24. Welschen LM, Bloemendal E, Nijpels G, Dekker JM, Heine RJ, Stalman WA, Bouter LM. Self-monitoring of blood glucose in patients with type 2 diabetes who are not using insulin. *Cochrane Database Syst Rev* 2005; Issue 2: Art. no. CD005060.

25. Cappuccio FP, Kerry SM, Forbes L, Donald A. Blood pressure control by home monitoring: meta-analysis of randomised trials. *BMJ* 2004;329(7458):145.

26. Louis AA, Turner T, Gretton M, Baksh A, Cleland JG. A systematic review of telemonitoring for the management of heart failure. *Eur J Heart Fail* 2003;5(5): 583–590.

27. Kelham CL. Self-monitoring of blood pressure at home: informed self-regulation of drug treatment could be next step. *BMJ* 2005;330(7483):148.

28. Gibson PG, Powell H, Coughlan J, Wilson AJ, Abramson M, Haywood P, *et al.* Self-management education and regular practitioner review for adults with asthma. *Cochrane Database Syst Rev* 2003; Issue 1: Art. no. CD001117.

29. Balas EA, Jaffrey F, Kuperman GJ, Boren SA, Brown GD, Pinciroli F, Mitchell JA. Electronic communication with patients: evaluation of distance medicine technology. *JAMA* 1997;278(2):152–159.

30. Wallace P, Haines A, Harrison R, Barber J, Thompson S, Jacklin P, Roberts J, Lewis L, Wainwright P, Virtual Outreach Project Group. Joint teleconsultations (virtual outreach) versus standard outpatient appointments for patients referred by their general practitioner for a specialist opinion: a randomised trial. *Lancet* 2002; 359(9322): 1961–1968.

31. Healthgrid.org. The Healthgrid White Paper. http://www.healthgrid.org (accessed on 14 July 2005).

32. Yamey G. Medicines Control Agency takes over GP research database. *BMJ* 1999;319:1153.

33. The General Practice Research Database (GPRD) and Academic Research. http:// www.gprd.com/academia/ (accessed on 13 July 2005).

34. Cleary P, Shorvon S, Tallis R. Late-onset seizures as a predictor of subsequent stroke. *Lancet* 2004;363(9416):1184–1186.

35. Rector A, Taweel A, Rogers J, Ingram D, Kalra D, Gaizauskas R, Hepple M, Milan J, Powers R, Scott D, Singleton P. Joining up health and bioinformatics: e-Science meets e-Health. Proceedings of the All-Hands Meeting 2004. http://www. allhands.org.uk/2004/proceedings/papers/118.pdf (accessed on 13 July 2005).

36. Humphreys K, Demetriou G, Gaizauskas R. Bioinformatics applications of information extraction from journal articles. *J Inf Sci* 2000;26(2):75–85.

Index